Application of
Nursing Process
and
Nursing Diagnosis:
An Interactive Text for
Diagnostic Reasoning

Application of Nursing Process and Nursing Diagnosis:

An Interactive Text for Diagnostic Reasoning
second edition

Marilynn E. Doenges, RN, BSN, MA, CS
Clinical Specialist
Adult Psychiatric/Mental Health Nursing
Private Practice
Instructor
Beth-El College of Nursing
Colorado Springs, Colorado

Mary Frances Moorhouse, RN, CCP, CCRN, CRRN
Nurse Consultant
TNT-RN Enterprises
Colorado Springs, Colorado

Joseph T. Burley, RN, MNED
College of Nursing
University of Florida
Gainesville, Florida

 F. A. DAVIS COMPANY • Philadelphia

F. A. Davis Company
1915 Arch Street
Philadelphia, PA 19103

Printed in the United States of America

Last digit indicates print number: 10 9 8 7 6 5 4 3 2

Publisher: Robert Martone
Nursing Developmental Editor: Melanie Freely
Production Editor: Marianne Fithian
Cover Designer: Louis J. Forgione

As new scientific information becomes available through basic and clinical research, recommended treatments and drug therapies undergo changes. The author(s) and publisher have done everything possible to make this book accurate, up to date, and in accord with accepted standards at the time of publication. The authors, editors, and publisher are not responsible for errors or omissions or for consequences from application of the book, and make no warranty, expressed or implied, in regard to the contents of the book. Any practice described in this book should be applied by the reader in accordance with professional standards of care used in regard to the unique circumstances that may apply in each situation. The reader is advised always to check product information (package inserts) for changes and new information regarding dose and contraindications before administering any drug. Caution is especially urged when using new or infrequently ordered drugs.

Library of Congress Cataloging-in-Publication Data

Doenges, Marilynn E., 1922–
    Application of nursing process and nursing diagnosis : an
interactive text for diagnostic reasoning / Marilynn E. Doenges,
Mary Frances Moorhouse, Joseph Burley. — 2nd ed.
        p.   cm.
    Includes bibliographical references and index.
    ISBN 0-8036-2676-2
    1. Nursing.   2. Nursing assessment.   3. Nursing diagnosis.
4. Nursing records.   I. Moorhouse, Mary Frances, 1947–   .
II. Burley, Joseph T.   III. Title.
    [DNLM: 1. Nursing Process.   2. Nursing Diagnosis—methods. WY
100 D615a 1995]
RT41.D54 1995
610.73 — dc20
DNLM/DLC
for Library of Congress   94-47073
                                                                    CIP

To our families, who support us in all we do and who continue to support our dreams, fantasies, and obsessions:

With special thanks to:

our spouses, Dean, Jan, and Jolene;

our children and grandchildren,

Nancy, Jim, Jennifer, and Jonathan Daigle; David, Monita, Matthew, and Tyler Doenges; Jim Doenges; Barbara Doenges, and Bob Lanza; John, Holly, Nicole, and Kelsey Doenges; Paul Moorhouse; Jason, Ellaina, and Alexa Moorhouse; Joel and Justin Burley;

Alice Geissler, for being available when we need help;

The staff at Memorial Hospital library, for cheerfuly filling in all the blanks and patiently helping us find those elusive references.

To the students of Beth-El College of Nursing and the students of the College of Nursing, University of Florida, who continue to challenge us to make the nursing process and nursing diagnosis understandable.

To our colleagues, who continue to provide a sounding board and feedback for our professional beliefs and expectations. We hope this interactive text will help you and your students at all stages to clarify and apply these concepts.

Kudos to the F. A. Davis staff,

To our publisher and friend Robert (Bob) Martone;

To Ruth DeGeorge, who has shown great patience and served as a buffer for all involved;

To Melanie Freely, Herb Powell, and Marianne Fithian who facilitated the revision process to get this project completed in a timely fashion.

Lastly, to the nurses who have patiently awaited this revision, we hope it will help in applying theory to practice and enhance the delivery and effectiveness of your care.

Notes To The Educator

The nursing process has been used for over 25 years as a systematic approach to nursing practice. The process is both an efficient and effective method for organizing nursing knowledge and clinical decision making in providing planned patient care. Although it has been undergoing constant reevaluation and revision, the concepts within the process still remain central to nursing practice.

Healthcare accrediting agencies and nursing organizations have developed standards of nursing practice that focus on the tenets of the nursing process—that is, assessing, diagnosing, planning, implementing, evaluating, and documenting patient care. Although, the formats used to document the plan of care may change with the interpretation and evaluation of standards, the nursing responsibilities and interventions required for planned patient care still need to be learned, shared, performed, evaluated, and documented.

The nursing process is by its nature an interactive method of practicing nursing. This text mirrors that interactive focus by presenting a step-by-step problem-solving design to help students develop an understanding of the meaning and language of nursing. We have included definitions and professional standards that will serve as a solid foundation for your students to understand and apply the nursing process. These activities encourage the student to actively seek solutions rather than passively assimilate knowledge. The vignettes, practice activities, work pages, and case studies provide an opportunity to examine and scrutinize patient situations and dilemmas in practice, consider alternatives, and evaluate outcomes. The worksheets serve as graphic summaries that provide students with criteria to evaluate their decisions and demonstrate their understanding of the concepts and integration of the material presented. Tear-out pages for independent learning provide an opportunity for practical application and beginning mastery of the nursing process. These pages can be taken to the clinical area to reinforce selected aspects of the nursing process. Finally, review of patient situations and the Code for Nurses can serve as a catalyst for philosophical and ethical discussions that can stimulate critical thinking.

CHAPTER 1, THE NURSING PROCESS: DELIVERING QUALITY CARE

This introductory chapter presents an overview of the nursing process. Students are introduced to the definitions of nursing and nursing diagnosis and the American Nurses Association's Standards of Clinical Nursing Practice.

CHAPTER 2, THE ASSESSMENT STEP: DEVELOPING THE PATIENT DATA BASE

This chapter gives the students their introduction to the first step of the nursing process. Organizational formats for constructing nursing assessment tools are discussed and both the physical and psychosocial aspects of assessment are blended into the interview process. Examples of patient data assist students to identify categories of nursing diagnostic labels.

CHAPTER 3, PROBLEM IDENTIFICATION STEP: ANALYZING THE DATA

The definition and concepts of nursing diagnosis are presented in this chapter. We use the term *Patient Diagnostic Statement* to describe the combination of the NANDA-approved label, the patient's related factors (etiology), and associated defining characteristics (signs/symptoms). A six-step diagnostic reasoning process is presented to assist students in their beginning efforts to accurately analyze the patient's assessment data. The remainder of this chapter focuses on ruling-out, synthesizing, evaluating, and constructing the patient diagnostic statement.

CHAPTER 4, THE PLANNING STEP: CREATING THE PLAN OF CARE

Information on developing the individualized outcomes for the patient is provided in this chapter. A focus on correctly writing measurable outcomes is initially presented. Nursing interventions are defined and acknowledgment of the work by the Iowa Intervention Project's Nursing Interventions Classification (NIC) is included. The topics, priorities of interventions, discharge planning, and selecting appropriate nursing interventions are discussed. A practice activity for recording the steps of the nursing process learned thus far is included to provide the student a realistic application. An interactive plan of care worksheet is used to present examples and guidelines for developing the patient's outcome statement, selecting nursing interventions, and providing rationales for nursing interventions.

CHAPTER 5, THE IMPLEMENTATION STEP: PUTTING THE PLAN OF CARE INTO ACTION

Information is presented about the validation and implementation of the plan of care. Concerns regarding the day-to-day organization of the nurse's work is creatively used in a practice activity where students use time management to plan the day's patient care interventions. Change-of-shift reporting principles are also discussed and practiced.

CHAPTER 6, THE EVALUATION STEP: DETERMINING WHETHER DESIRED OUTCOMES HAVE BEEN MET

The crucial step of evaluation and its accompanying reassessment and revision processes are presented in this chapter on the last step of the nursing process. A practice activity is provided to help students evaluate the plan of care partially constructed in Chapter 4. Revisions to the plan of care are necessary and the activity provides a realistic exercise for this final step. The interactive plan of care worksheet is designed to ask your students questions about their patient's progress and the effectiveness of their implemented nursing interventions.

CHAPTER 7, DOCUMENTING THE NURSING PROCESS

This chapter introduces students to ways of successfully documenting their use of the nursing process. Communication, legal responsibilities, and reimbursement are a few of the topics introduced in this chapter. The documentation systems of SOAP and FOCUS Charting™ are presented to depict two possible methods of documenting the nursing process. The last section of the interactive worksheet focuses the students' attention on three important aspects of documentation: the reassessment data, interventions implemented, and the patient's response.

CHAPTER 8, INTERACTIVE CARE PLANNING: FROM ASSESSMENT TO PATIENT RESPONSE

This final chapter provides an evaluation checklist that can be used to evaluate your students' progress in all aspects of the nursing process. The checklist is designed to include the criteria listed on the Interactive Care Plan Worksheets, ANA Standards of Clinical Nursing Practice, and the JCAHO nursing standards. The chapter ends with a case study that gives your students an opportunity to apply all the steps of the nursing process. The evaluation checklist along with the TIME OUTS included in the plan of care worksheets provide the students with the required guidance when constructing their first complete plan of care.

APPENDICES

A listing of the North American Nursing Diagnosis Association nursing diagnoses are included in Appendix A. Each nursing diagnosis' definition, related/risk factors, and defining characteristics are provided to assist the student in accurately selecting the appropriate nursing diagnosis.

Appendix B provides an adult medical-surgical assessment tool as referenced in Chapter 2 along with excerpts from assessment tools developed for the psychiatric and obstetrical settings. The tools are helpful in assisting students in assessing the patient's response to health problems as well as gathering physical assessment data.

Appendix C organizes the NANDA diagnostic labels within Maslow's hierarchy of needs to aid in visualizing and determining priorities for providing patient care.

Appendix D, Code for Nurses, was included for your use in both the classroom and during clinical rounds to share with your students the values that guide nursing practice today. A reference to the Code and the introduction of a discussion of beliefs that affect nursing practice are contained in Chapter 1 and an ethical activity is presented in Chapter 5.

Appendices E and F provide tools for the student to measure the accuracy of their choice of nursing diagnosis labels. The Ordinal Scale of Accuracy of a Nursing Diagnosis assigns a point value to a diagnosis that is consistent with the number of cues and disconfirming cues identified. This tool aids the student in validating their analysis of the collected data and choice of nursing diagnosis. The Integrated Model for Self-Monitoring of the Diagnostic Process provides direct feedback to students but can also be shared with you to demonstrate the students progress in data analysis and diagnosis.

Appendix G is a sample of a Clinical (Critical) Pathway, providing you the opportunity to address alternate forms for planning and evaluating care.

Appendix H presents some commonly accepted charting abbreviations, which may be useful in your discussion of the documentation process.

Finally Appendix I and J are the Keys to the Learning Activities provided in the text.

The National League for Nursing emphasizes the need for graduates of nursing programs to think critically, make decisions, and formulate independent judgments. To achieve this outcome, you as an instructor are encouraged to use teaching strategies that will "stimulate higher-order critical thinking in both theory and practice situations" (Klaassens, 1988). These strategies include: questioning, analysis, synthesis, application, writing, problem-solving games, and philosophical discussions.

It is our hope that the interactive features of this text will provide the strategies to assist you in successfully sharing with your students the meaning and language of the nursing process and in making a smooth and effective transition from the classroom to any clinical setting.

Marilynn E. Doenges
Mary Frances Moorhouse
Joseph T. Burley

Notes To The Student

The nursing process will be described by your instructors as a systematic approach to the practice of nursing. You will shortly find that this process is an efficient and effective method for organizing both nursing knowledge and practice. The process will also assist you in accurately performing clinical decision making activities in planning your patient's care. The process has been continually refined since its inception in the 1960s. However, to date, the concepts within the process still remain central to nursing practice. Through the use of this text your instructors will share the meaning of the concepts and this evolving nursing practice language with you.

The nursing process is an interactive method of practicing nursing with the components fitting together in a continuous cycle of thought and action. This interactive focus was used in developing and writing this text for you. The text focuses on the steps of the nursing process and provides information and exercises to aid your understanding and application of the process. Included are practice activities, ongoing reference to simulated clinical experiences through the use of vignettes, and end of chapter work pages to promote your understanding. Definitions of both nursing and the nursing process along with the American Nurses Association's (ANA) Standards of Clinical Nursing Practice are presented to provide a solid foundation for you to build an understanding of the language and knowledge of nursing and application of the nursing process.

In addition, a six-step diagnostic reasoning/critical thinking process is presented for accurately analyzing the patient's assessment data. It will assist you in ruling out, synthesizing, evaluating, and constructing the patient diagnostic statement, which is pivotal for developing individualized plans of care for your patients. A practice activity for writing a nursing plan of care was developed to provide a realistic application of your newly learned knowledge. An example of a typical day's work requirements is used in a practice activity where you are given the opportunity to use time management principles and skills to plan your patient's care within an 8-hour shift. A third practice activity is provided to give you a chance to choose patient information you would include in a change-of-shift report to communicate the outcomes of your use of the nursing process.

Next, you are given an opportunity to test your beginning skills in developing a complete plan of care. A set of step-by-step forms are provided for you to document your clinical judgment by selecting two patient diagnostic statements, developing the goals/outcomes, and identifying the nursing interventions. Finally, an evaluation checklist is provided to serve as a valuable self-assessment of the appropriateness and accuracy of your comprehension of the planning exercise and future plans of care that you will design for your patients.

At the end of the chapters, a bibliography and list of suggested reading are included to guide you in further and future reading and understanding of both nursing knowledge and nursing process. In Chapter 1, a suggested reading list provides a listing of publications from a historical perspective. The listing should be helpful to you in searching out the meaning of nursing and the nursing process. The list may also prove valuable in writing varied required papers on similar topics. Use and enjoy. The second section gives you the most current listing of publications at the time of the printing of this second edition. Once again, the selected publications are provided to assist you in this learning process.

The perforated tear-out pages for the end of chapter work pages, interactive care plan worksheets, and the evaluation checklist were especially designed for your independent learning. These tear-out pages can be taken to the clinical area to reinforce selected aspects of the nursing process. It is our hope that the interactive features of this text will assist you in making the successful and effective transition from the classroom to your assigned clinical setting. We wish you well in this beginning phase of your new profession.

Marilynn E. Doenges
Mary Frances Moorhouse
Joseph T. Burley

Acknowledgments

To Alice Geissler, RN, BSN, CCRN
Colorado Springs, Colorado

To Jean Jenny, MS, MEd, BScNEd, RN
Former Professor
Faculty of Health Sciences
University of Ottowa
School of Nursing
Ottowa, Ontario
Canada

To Barbara Ogden, RN, MSN
Assistant Professor
College of Nursing
University of Florida
Gainesville, Florida
a mentor, colleague, and friend. Thank you.

To Paladin Productions
whose computer talents clarified our ideas and made them visible.

Contents

Practice Activities and Work Pages

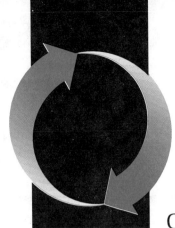

The Nursing Process: Delivering Quality Care

- ■ The Nursing Profession
- ■ The Nursing Process
- ■ How the Nursing Process Works
- ■ Practice Advantages of the Nursing Process
- ■ Summary

THE NURSING PROFESSION

Nursing is both a science and an art concerned with the physical, psychological, sociological, cultural, and spiritual concerns of the individual. The science of nursing is based on a broad theoretical framework; its art is dependent on the caring skills and abilities of the individual nurse. The importance of the nurse within the healthcare system is being recognized in many positive ways, and the profession of nursing is itself acknowledging the need for its practitioners to be professional and accountable.

In its early developmental years, nursing did not seek or have the means to control its own practice. Florence Nightingale, in discussing the nature of nursing, observed that "nursing has been limited to signify little more than the administration of medicines and the application of poultices" (Nightingale, 1859). Although this attitude has persisted into the present, the nursing profession has been working to define what makes nursing unique and to identify its body of professional knowledge.

Thus, barely a century after Miss Nightingale noted that "the very elements of nursing are all but unknown," the American Nurses' Association

DEFINITION
OF NURSING

*Nursing is the diagnosis
and treatment of
human responses to
health and illness (ANA,
1987).*

(ANA) developed the ANA Social Policy Statement (1980) defining nursing as "the diagnosis and treatment of human responses to actual or potential health problems." In ANA's Scope of Nursing Practice (1987) a broader definition was suggested: "Nursing is the diagnosis and treatment of human responses to health and illness." In the modern world of nursing, therefore, human responses, defined as people's experiences with and responses to health and illness, are the phenomena of concern for nurses. Thus, nursing's role includes health promotion as well as activities that contribute to recovery from or adjustment to illness. Also, nurses support the right of patients to define their own health-related goals and engage in care that reflects their values.

THE NURSING PROCESS

DEFINITION
OF NURSING
PROCESS

*The nursing process is a
five-step process:*

1. *Nursing Assessment*

2. *Problem Identifica-
tion/Analysis (nurs-
ing diagnosis)*

3. *Planning*

4. *Implementation*

5. *Evaluation*

*The nursing process
provides an orderly,
logical problem-solving
approach for adminis-
tering nursing care so
that the patient's needs
for such care are met
comprehensively and
effectively.*

Nursing leaders have identified a process that "combines the most desirable elements of the art of nursing with the most relevant elements of systems theory, using the scientific method" (Shore, 1988). This process incorporates an interactive/interpersonal approach with a problem-solving and decision-making process (Peplau, 1952; Travelbee, 1971; King, 1971; Yura & Walsh, 1988).

The nursing process was first introduced in the 1950s as a three-step process of assessment, planning, and evaluation based on the scientific method of observing, measuring, gathering data, and analyzing the findings. Years of study, use, and refinement have led nurses to expand the nursing process to five distinct steps which provide an efficient method of organizing thought processes for clinical decision making, problem solving, and delivery of higher quality, individualized patient care. Box 1–1 shows the steps and their order. These five steps are central to nursing actions in any setting. The nursing process is now included in the conceptual framework of nursing curricula and is accepted as part of the legal definition of nursing in the Nurse Practice Acts of most states.

When a patient enters the healthcare system, the steps of the nursing process are set into motion. The nurse collects data, identifies patient problems/needs (nursing diagnoses), establishes goals, identifies outcomes, and se-

---

BOX 1–1 STEPS OF THE NURSING PROCESS

The nursing process consists of five specific steps:

1. *Assessment:* A systematic collection of data relating to patients.
2. *Problem Identification:* Analysis of collected data to identify the patient's problems and needs.
3. *Planning:* A two-part process: first the identification of goals and the patient's desired outcomes to correct the assessed health problem or need, and second, the selection of appropriate nursing interventions to assist the patient in attaining the outcomes.
4. *Implementation:* Putting the plan of care into action.
5. *Evaluation:* Determining the patient's progress toward attaining the identified outcome, and the patient's response to and effectiveness of the selected nursing interventions. Then changing the plan if indicated.

lects nursing interventions to assist the patient in achieving these outcomes and goals. Finally, after these interventions have been implemented, the nurse evaluates the patient's responses and the effectiveness of the plan of care in reaching the desired outcomes and goals to determine whether or not the problems have been resolved and the patient is ready to be discharged from the care setting. If the identified problems remain unresolved, further assessment, additional problem identification, alteration of outcomes and goals, and/or changes of interventions are required.

Although we use the terms *assessment, problem identification, planning, implementation*, and *evaluation* as separate, progressive steps, in reality they are interrelated. Together these steps form a continuous circle of thought and action, which recycles throughout the patient's contact with the healthcare system. Figure 1–1 shows a model of how this cycling process can be visualized. You can see that the nursing process uses the skills of critical thinking and creates a method of active problem solving that is both dynamic and cyclic.

HOW THE NURSING PROCESS WORKS

The scientific method of problem solving introduced in the previous section is used almost instinctively by most people, without conscious awareness, as noted in Box 1–2. Because the nursing process is based on this method, it may seem somewhat familiar. You will only need to learn the new terms required by the nursing process, rather than having to think about each step (assessment, problem identification, planning, implementation, and evaluation) in an entirely new way.

To effectively use the nursing process, there are some basic abilities that the nurse must possess and be able to apply. Particularly important is a thorough knowledge of science and theory, not only as applied in nursing, but

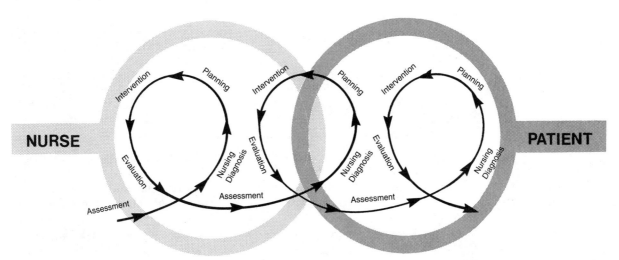

Figure 1–1. Diagram of the nursing process. The steps of the nursing process are interrelated, forming a continuous circle of throught and action that is both dynamic and cyclic.

BOX 1–2   PROBLEM SOLVING: EVERYDAY USE OF THE NURSING PROCESS

You have celebrated completion of your semester finals with a very spicy, late evening dinner. You awaken during the night with a burning sensation in the center of your chest. You are young and in good health and note no other symptoms (*Assessment*). You decide that your pain is the result of the spicy food you have eaten (*Problem Identification*). You then determine that you need to relieve the discomfort before you will be able to return to sleep (*Planning*). You take a liquid antacid for your discomfort (*Implementation*). Within a few minutes, you note the burning sensation is relieved, and you return to bed without further concern (*Evaluation*).

This is a process you routinely use to solve problems in your own life that can be readily applied to patient-care situations.

---

also in other related disciplines such as medicine and psychology. Creativity is needed in the application of nursing knowledge, as well as adaptability in handling change and the many unexpected happenings that occur. As a nurse, you must make a commitment to practice your profession in the best possible way, trusting in yourself and your ability to do your job well and displaying the necessary leadership to organize and supervise as your position requires. In addition, intelligence, well-developed interpersonal skills, and competent technical skills are essential.

> **For example:** A patient's irritable behavior could be a sign of anger or it could arise from a sense of helplessness regarding life events. However, it could also be the result of low blood glucose or the effects of excessive caffeine intake. A single behavior may have varied causes. It is important that your nursing assessment skills identify the underlying etiology to provide appropriate care.

BOX 1–3   FUNDAMENTAL PHILOSOPHICAL BELIEFS IN NURSING

There are several fundamental philosophical beliefs that are essential to the practice of nursing and need to be kept in mind when using the nursing process:

- The patient is a human being who has worth and dignity.
- There are basic human needs that must be met   (see Chapter 2, Maslow's Hierarchy).
- When these needs are not met, problems arise that may require intervention by another person until the individual can resume responsibility for themselves.
- Patients have a right to quality health and nursing care delivered with interest, compassion, and competence with a focus on wellness and prevention.
- The therapeutic nurse-patient relationship is important in this process.

In addition to these abilities, there are several fundamental beliefs (Box 1–3) that provide guidance for the application of the nursing process and enhance the quality of nursing care. To further increase your knowledge and clinical decision-making skills, Appendix D contains the 11 statements of the ANA Code for Nurses (ANA, 1985). We suggest you take the time to read, think about, and incorporate these 11 statements into your professional practice and refer to the complete work for interpretation of the code statements.

The practice responsibilities presented in the definitions of nursing and the nursing process are explained in detail in the publication, *Standards of Clinical Nursing Practice* (1991). The standards provide workable guidelines to ensure that the practice of nursing can be carried out by each individual nurse. Table 1–1 presents an abbreviated description of the standards of clinical practice. With the ultimate goal of quality health care, the effective use of the nursing process will result in a viable nursing-care system that is recognized and accepted as nursing's body of knowledge and that can be shared with other healthcare professionals.

Table 1–1 ANA STANDARDS OF CLINICAL NURSING PRACTICE

Standards of Care

Describes a competent level of nursing care as demonstrated by the nursing process that encompasses all significant actions taken by the nurse in providing care, and forms the foundation of clinical decision making.

1. **Assessment:** the nurse collects client health data.
2. **Diagnosis:** the nurse analyzes the assessment data in determining diagnoses.
3. **Outcome Identification:** the nurse identifies expected outcomes individualized to the client.
4. **Planning:** the nurse develops a plan of care that prescribes interventions to attain expected outcomes.
5. **Implementation:** the nurse implements the interventions identified in the plan of care.
6. **Evaluation:** the nurse evaluates the client's progress toward attainment of outcomes.

Standards of Professional Performance

Describes roles expected of all professional nurses appropriate to their education, position, and practice setting.

1. **Quality of Care:** the nurse systematically evaluates the quality and effectiveness of nursing practice.
2. **Performance Appraisal:** the nurse evaluates his/her own nursing practice in relation to professional practice standards and relevant statutes and regulations.
3. **Education:** the nurse acquires and maintains current knowledge in nursing practice.
4. **Collegiality:** the nurse contributes to the professional development of peers, colleagues, and others.
5. **Ethics:** the nurse's decisions and actions on behalf of clients are determined in an ethical manner.
6. **Collaboration:** the nurse collaborates with the client, significant others, and healthcare providers in providing client care.
7. **Research:** the nurse uses research findings in practice.
8. **Resource Utilization:** the nurse considers factors related to safety, effectiveness, and cost in planning and delivering client care.

PRACTICE ADVANTAGES OF THE NURSING PROCESS

There are many advantages to the use of the nursing process:

- The nursing process provides a framework for meeting the individual needs of the patient, the patient's family/significant other(s), and the community.
- The steps of the nursing process focus the nurse's attention on the "individual" human responses of a patient/group to a given health situation, resulting in a holistic plan of care addressing their specific problems/needs.
- The nursing process provides an organized, systematic method of problem solving, which may minimize dangerous errors or omissions in caregiving, and avoid time-consuming repetition in care and documentation.
- The use of the nursing process promotes the active involvement of the patient in his or her own health care, enhancing consumer satisfaction. Such participation increases the patient's sense of control over what is happening to him or her, stimulates problem solving, and promotes personal responsibility, all of which strengthen the patient's commitment to achieving identified goals.
- The use of the nursing process enables you as a nurse to have more control over your own practice. This enhances the opportunity for you to use your knowledge, expertise, and intuition constructively and dynamically to increase the likelihood of a successful patient outcome. This, in turn, promotes greater job satisfaction and professional growth.
- The use of the nursing process provides a common language for practice, unifying the nursing profession. Using a system that clearly communicates the plan of care to coworkers and patients enhances continuity of care, promotes achievement of patient goals, provides a vehicle for evaluation, and aids in the development of nursing standards. In addition, the structure of the process provides a format for documenting the patient's response to all aspects of the planned care.
- The use of the nursing process provides a means of assessing nursing's economic contribution to patient care. The nursing process supplies a vehicle for the quantitative and qualitative measurement of nursing care that meets the goal of cost effectiveness and still promotes holistic care.

SUMMARY

In using the nursing process to administer nursing care to patients, the nursing profession has identified a body of knowledge that contributes to the prevention of illness as well as to the maintenance and/or restoration of the patient's health (or relief of pain/discomfort and provision of support when a return to health is not possible). The nursing process is the basis of all nursing actions and is the essence of nursing. It can be applied in any healthcare or educational setting, in any theoretical or conceptual framework, and within the context of any nursing philosophy. The process is flexible and yet sufficiently structured to provide a base for nursing actions.

The following chapters will identify, discuss, and clarify each step of the nursing process. As noted, each step of the process builds on and interacts with the other steps ensuring an effective practice model. Inclusion of the standards of clinical nursing practice in the appropriate chapters will provide additional information to reinforce your understanding and opportunities to apply your knowledge by means of Practice Activities and a Work Page at the end of each chapter. Four patients will be helping you in your learning process by sharing their personal experiences:

- Robert is a 72-year-old male admitted to a medical inpatient unit for a recurrence of bilateral lower lobe pneumonia. He is a retired truck driver living alone since his wife's death 5 years ago. He is concerned about his future and about losing control of his life, which will present you with ethical concerns and challenges in dealing with family dynamics.

- Sally is a 30-year-old female who is pregnant and experiencing beginning labor. This is her third pregnancy. Sally completed her evening shift as a respiratory therapist although she noted early signs of labor at 8:00 PM You will be able to follow Sally through labor, delivery, and home visits by a public health nurse to enhance your understanding of the continuity of care.

- Michelle, a 14-year-old female, has suffered multiple injuries in a mountain bike accident. She is a ninth grader at the local high school and lives with her parents, an older brother, and a younger sister. You will find pain management a major aspect of your nursing interventions for Michelle.

- Donald, a 46-year-old male, is being treated for depression after the loss of his position as a loan banker because of his chronic absenteeism and poor job performance related to alcohol abuse. He has been drinking heavily recently and is suffering alcohol withdrawal since his admission. You will follow Donald through his other assessed healthcare needs of nutrition, coping, and changes in his role expectations.

The use of these vignettes will provide many clinical examples throughout the text, offering a simulated practice environment and a touch of reality in planning the required continuity of patient care.

Two suggested reading lists are included at the end of this first chapter to assist you in your journey of understanding the historical development of the nursing process and to become knowledgeable about current publications describing these topics. We suggest that sometime during your busy program you take the time to read and reflect on these early authors' meaning and the language of nursing and the nursing process.

WORK PAGE: Chapter One

1. The ANA has defined nursing as: the diagnosis + treatment of human responses to health + illness.

2. My own definition of nursing is: someone who helps the sick people to become well and who teaches all people benefits of wellness.

3. How has the information in this chapter affected your definition? It has taught me that there are guidlines to help me diagnose.

4. The ANA Social Policy Statement defines the phenomena of concern for nurses as: the diagnoses and treatment of human responses to actual or potential health problems.

5. The definition of nursing process is: an orderly logical problem-solving approach for administering nursing care so that the patients needs for such care are met comprehensively + effectively.

6. Name and define the five steps of the nursing process and provide an example of each step:

Steps	Definition	Example
a. Assessment	a systematic collection of data relating to patients	someone young in good health w/ no symptoms
b. Problem Identification	Analysis of collected data to identify the patients' problems + needs	pain resulting from spicy foods
c. Planning	developing a plan of care that prescribes interventions to attain expected outcomes	relieve discomfort
d. Implementation	putting the plan of care into action	take a liquid antacid
e. Evaluation	evaluating the clients progress toward attainment of outcomes	burning sensation relieved

7. List three advantages of using the nursing process:
   a. Provides a framework for meeting the individual needs of the patient, the patient's family | significant others, + the community.
   b. Steps focus the nurse's attention on the "individual" human responses of a patient/group to a given health situation, resulting in a holistic plan of care addressing their specific problems/needs.
   c. Provides an organized, systematic method of problem solving, which may minimize dangerous errors or omissions in caregiving, + avoid time-consuming repetition of care + documentation.

8. List two of the fundamental philosophical beliefs that you believe are basic to decision making within the nursing process:

a. _The patient is a human being who has worth + dignity._

b. _There are basic human needs that must be met._

9. Identify the steps of the nursing process by placing the appropriate number of the activity in the space following the data presented in the following vignette:
1 = Assessment; 2 = Problem identification;
3 = Planning; 4 = Implementation; 5 = Evaluation.

Vignette: Robert, a 72-year-old male, is admitted with recurrent bilateral lower lobe pneumonia. _____1_____

He reports this is his second episode in 6 months. __1__

Temperature is 101°F, skin hot and flushed. __1__

He reports frequent, hacking cough with moderate amount of thick greenish mucus. __1__

Auscultation of the chest reveals scattered rhonchi throughout. __21__

His mucous membranes are pale, and his lips are dry and cracked. __1__

He says when he was sick last month, the doctor prescribed an antibiotic which he discontinued after 6 days because he was feeling better. __1__

You determine Robert has an airway clearance problem, a fluid volume deficit, and is not managing his therapeutic regimen effectively and thus requires teaching to promote adequate self-care and to prevent recurrence. __2__

You establish the following outcomes:

- Expectorates secretions completely with breath sounds clear and respiration noiseless. __2__

- Demonstrates adequate fluid balance with moist mucous membranes and loose respiratory secretions. __2__

- Verbalizes understanding of cause of condition and rationale for therapeutic regimen. __3__

You decide to set up a regular schedule for respiratory activities and fluid replacement. __3__

In addition, you formulate a teaching plan to cover the identified concerns for self-care and illness prevention. __3__

You provide a tube of petroleum jelly for Robert to use on his lips. __4__

Every 2 hours you visit Robert to encourage him to deep-breathe, cough, change his position, and drink a glass of fluid of his choice. __4__

You use this time to discuss avoidance of crowds and individuals with upper respiratory infections and recommend continuing the treatment plan after discharge. __4__

The following day, Robert's skin is no longer hot and flushed, temperature is 99°F, secretions are loose and readily expectorated, and breath sounds are clearing. __5__

Robert's lips and oral mucous membranes are moist. He is able to explain in his own words how to care for himself and how to prevent pneumonia. __5__

You decide that the current treatment plan is achieving the identified outcomes and to continue the plan as written. __5__

BIBLIOGRAPHY

American Nurses' Association. (1980). *Nursing: A Social Policy Statement.* Kansas City, MO: Author.

American Nurses' Association. (1985). *Code for Nurses With Interpretive Statements.* Kansas City, MO: Author.

American Nurses' Association. (1987). *The Scope of Nursing Practice.* Kansas City, MO: Author.

American Nurses' Association. (1990). *Suggested State Legislation: Nursing Practice Act, Nursing Disciplinary Act, Prescriptive Authority Act.* Kansas City, MO: Author.

American Nurses' Association. (1991). *Standards of Clinical Nursing Practice.* Kansas City, MO: Author.

Barnum, B.S. (1990). *Nursing Theory: Analysis, Application, Evaluation* (3rd ed.). Glenview, IL: Scott, Foresman/Little, Brown.

Bulechek, G.M., & McCloskey, J.C. (Eds.). (1992). *Nursing Interventions: Essential Nursing Treatments* (2nd ed.). Philadelphia: W.B. Saunders.

King, L. (1971). *Toward a Theory for Nursing: General Concepts of Human Behavior.* New York: Wiley.

Nightingale, F. (1859). *Notes on Nursing: What It Is and What It Is Not* (Facsimile edition). Philadelphia: J.B. Lippincott, 1946.

North American Nursing Diagnosis Association. (1990). *Taxonomy I—Revised 1990: With Official Nursing Diagnoses.* St. Louis, MO: Author.

Peplau, H.E. (1952). *Interpersonal Relations in Nursing: A Conceptual Frame of Reference for Psychodynamic Nursing.* New York: Putnam.

Shore, L.S. (1988). *Nursing Diagnosis: What It Is and How to Do It, a Programmed Text.* Richmond, VA: Medical College of Virginia Hospitals.

Travelbee, J. (1971). *Interpersonal Aspects of Nursing* (2nd ed.). Philadelphia: F.A. Davis.

Yura, H., & Walsh, M.B. (1988). *The Nursing Process: Assessing, Planning, Implementing, Evaluating* (5th ed.). Norwalk, CT: Appleton & Lange.

SUGGESTED READING

Classical Publications

American Nurses' Association. (1973). *Standards of Nursing Practice.* Kansas City, MO: Author.

Aspinall, M.J., & Tanner, C.A. (1981). *Decision Making for Patient Care: Applying the Nursing Process.* New York: Appleton-Century-Crofts.

Bloch, D. (1974). Some crucial terms in nursing: What do they really mean? *Nursing Outlook. 22*(11):669–694.

Carlson, J.H., Craft, C.A., & McGuire, A.D. (1982). *Nursing Diagnosis.* Philadelphia: W.B. Saunders.

Carnevali, D.L. (1983). Nursing Care Planning: Diagnosis and Management (3rd ed.). Philadelphia: J.B. Lippincott.

Little, D.E., & Carnevali, D.I. (1976). *Nursing Care Planning* (2nd ed.). Philadelphia: J.B. Lippincott.

Orem, D.E. (1971). *Nursing: Concepts of Practice.* New York: McGraw-Hill.

Orlando, I.J. (1961). *The Dynamic Nurse-Patient Relationship: Function, Process, and Principles.* New York: Putnam.

Patterson, J.G., & Zderad, L.T. (1976). *Humanistic Nursing.* New York: Wiley.

Wiedenbach, E. (1964). *Clinical Nursing: A Helping Art.* New York: Springer.

Yura, H., & Walsh, M.B. (Eds.). (1967). *The Nursing Process*. Washington, DC: Catholic University of America Press.

Current Publications

Bulechek, G.M., & McCloskey, J.C. (Eds)(1985). *Nursing interventions: Treatments for Nursing Diagnoses*. Philadelphia: W.B. Saunders.

Carnevali, D.L., Mitchell, P.H., Woods, N.F., & Tanner, C.A. (1984). *Diagnostic Reasoning in Nursing*. Philadelphia: J.B. Lippincott.

Carnevali, D.L., & Thomas, M.D. (1993). *Diagnostic Reasoning and Treatment Decision Making in Nursing*. Philadelphia: J.B. Lippincott.

Carpenito, L.J. (1993). *Nursing Diagnosis: Application to Clinical Practice* (5th ed.). Philadelphia: J.B. Lippincott.

Cox, H., et al. (1993). *Clinical Applications of Nursing Diagnosis: Adult Health, Child Health, Women's Health, Mental Health, and Home Health* (2nd ed.). Philadelphia: F.A. Davis.

Craft, M.J., & Denehy, J.A. (1990). *Nursing Interventions for Infants and Children*. Philadelphia: W.B. Saunders.

Gordon, M. (1987). *Nursing Diagnosis: Process and Application* (2nd ed.). New York: McGraw-Hill.

Hannah, K.J., Reimer, M., Mills, W.C., & Letourneau, S. (Eds.). (1987). *Clinical Judgment and Decision Making: The Future With Nursing Diagnosis*. New York: Wiley.

Leuner, J.D., Manton, A.M., Kelliher, D.B., Sullivan, S.P., & Doherty, M. (1990). *Mastering the Nursing Process: A Case Study Approach*. Philadelphia: F.A. Davis.

Maas, M., Buckwalter, K.C., & Hardy, M. (1991). *Nursing Diagnosis and Interventions for the Elderly*. Menlo Park, CA: Addison-Wesley.

McCloskey, J.C., & Bulechek, G.M. (Eds.). (1992). *Iowa Intervention Project: Nursing Interventions Classification (NIC)*. St. Louis, MO: Mosby–Year Book.

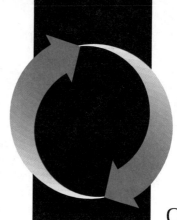

CHAPTER 2

The Assessment Step: Developing the Patient Data Base

ANA Standard 1: Assessment: *The nurse collects client health data.*

THE PATIENT DATA BASE

The ASSESSMENT step of the nursing process is an organized dynamic process involving three basic activities:

ASSESSMENT—the first step of the nursing process, during which data are collected.

13

- Systematically gathering data
- Sorting and organizing the data collected
- Documenting the data in a retrievable format

Using a number of techniques, you focus on eliciting a profile of the patient that will allow you to identify patient problems and corresponding nursing diagnoses, plan care, implement interventions, and evaluate outcomes. This profile is called the PATIENT DATA BASE, and it serves as the fundamental pool of knowledge about the patient from which all other steps of the nursing process proceed.

The patient data base supplies a sense of the patient's overall health status providing a picture of the patient's physical, psychological, sociocultural, spiritual, cognitive, developmental level, economic status, functional abilities, and lifestyle. It is a combination of data gathered from the history-taking interview (a method of obtaining SUBJECTIVE information by talking with the patient and/or significant other(s) and listening to their responses); the physical examination (a "hands-on" means of obtaining OBJECTIVE information); and data gathered from the results of *laboratory/diagnostic studies*. To be more specific, subjective data is what the patient/significant others perceive, and objective data is what you observe.

Because consistency is important, the same data collection model should be used for both the patient interview (history) and the physical examination, whether that model is a nursing framework, a systems approach, a head-to-toe approach, or a combination approach defined by your own agency. Frequently, to enhance efficiency and effectiveness, these two activities are combined into one interactive process in which physical data is gathered while interview questions are asked.

Framework for Data Collection

There are several nursing models that may be used to guide your data collection. Three of the commonly used models are shown in Table 2–1: Doenges and Moorhouse's Diagnostic Divisions, Gordon's Functional Health Patterns, and North American Nursing Diagnosis Association's (NANDA's) Human Response Patterns.

The use of a nursing model as a framework for data collection rather than a body systems approach (assessing the heart, moving on to the lungs) or the commonly known head-to-toe approach has the advantage of identifying and validating nursing diagnoses as opposed to MEDICAL DIAGNOSES. An assessment model such as the Assessment Tool shown in Appendix B limits repetitious collection of medical data, and focuses data collection on the nurse's phenomena of concern—the human responses to actual and potential health problems. Such responses include self-care limitations; impaired functioning in areas such as sleep, rest, nutrition, and elimination; pain; deficiencies in decision making, and problematic relationships (ANA, 1980).

The Interview Process

Information in the patient data base is obtained both from the patient and from family members/significant others (as appropriate) through conversation and by observation during a structured interview. The nursing interview may

PATIENT DATA BASE—the compilation of data collected about a patient; it consists of the nursing history, physical examination, and results of the diagnostic studies.

SUBJECTIVE DATA—what the patient reports, believes, or feels.

OBJECTIVE DATA—what can be observed, for example, vital signs, behaviors, diagnostic studies.

MEDICAL DIAGNOSIS—illnesses/conditions for which treatment is directed by a licensed physician; medical diagnoses focus on correction/prevention of the pathology of specific organs/body systems.

Table 2-1 **COMPARISON OF NURSING MODELS FOR DATA COLLECTION**

DIAGNOSTIC DIVISIONS (DOENGES AND MOORHOUSE, 1993)	FUNCTIONAL HEALTH PATTERNS (GORDON, 1993)	HUMAN RESPONSE PATTERNS (FITZPATRICK, 1991)
Activity/Rest: Ability to engage in necessary/desired activities of life (work and leisure) and to obtain adequate sleep/rest.	**Health Perception/Health Management:** Client's perception of general health status and well-being. Adherence to preventive health practices.	**Choosing:** To select between alternatives; the action of selecting or exercising preference in regard to a matter in which one is a free agent; to determine in favor of a course; to decide in accordance with inclinations.
Circulation: Ability to transport oxygen and nutrients necessary to meet cellular needs.	**Nutritional-Metabolic:** Patterns of food and fluid intake, fluid and electrolyte balance, general ability to heal.	**Communicating:** To converse; to impart, confer, or transmit thoughts, feelings, or information, internally or externally, verbally or nonverbally.
Ego Integrity: Ability to develop and use skills and behaviors to integrate and manage life experiences.	**Elimination:** Patterns of excretory function (bowel, bladder, and skin), and client's perception.	**Exchanging:** To give, relinquish or lose something while receiving something in return; the substitution of one element for another; the reciprocal act of giving and receiving.
Elimination: Ability to excrete waste products.	**Activity/Exercise:** Pattern of exercise, activity, leisure, recreation, and ADL; factors that interfere with desired or expected individual pattern.	
Food/Fluid: Ability to maintain intake of and use nutrients and liquids to meet physiologic needs.	**Cognitive-Perceptual:** Adequacy of sensory modes, such as vision, hearing, taste, touch, smell, pain perception, cognitive functional abilities.	**Feeling:** To experience, a consciousness, sensation, apprehension or sense; to be consciously or emotionally affected by a fact, event or state.
Hygiene: Ability to perform activities of daily living (ADL).	**Sleep/Rest:** Patterns of sleep and rest-relaxation periods during 24 hour day, as well as quality and quantity.	**Knowing:** To recognize or acknowledge a thing or a person; to be familiar with by experience or through information or report; to be cognizant of something through observation, inquiry or information; to be conversant with a body of facts, principles, or methods of action; to understand.
Neurosensory: Ability to perceive, integrate, and respond to internal and external cues.	**Self-Perception/Self-Concept:** Individual's attitudes about self, perception of abilities, body image, identity, general sense of worth and emotional patterns.	
Pain/Discomfort: Ability to control internal/external environment to maintain comfort.	**Role/Relationship:** Client's perception of major roles and responsibilities in current life situation.	**Moving:** To change the place or position of a body or any member of the body; to put and/or keep in motion; to provoke an excretion or discharge; the urge to action or to do something; to take action.
Respiration: Ability to provide and use oxygen to meet physiologic needs.	**Sexuality/Reproductive:** Client's perceived satisfaction or dissatisfaction with sexuality. Reproductive stage and pattern.	
Safety: Ability to provide safe, growth-promoting environment.	**Coping/Stress Tolerance:** General coping pattern, stress tolerance, support systems, and perceived ability to control and manage situations.	**Perceiving:** To apprehend with the mind; to become aware of by the senses; to apprehend what is not open or present to observation; to take fully or adequately.
Sexuality: (Component of Ego Integrity and Social Interaction) Ability to meet requirements/characteristics of male/female role.		
Social Interaction: Ability to establish and maintain relationships.		
Teaching/Learning: Ability to incorporate and use information to achieve healthy lifestyle/optimal wellness.		

(Continued)

Table 2–1   COMPARISON OF NURSING MODELS FOR DATA COLLECTION (Continued)

DIAGNOSTIC DIVISIONS (DOENGES AND MOORHOUSE, 1993)	FUNCTIONAL HEALTH PATTERNS (GORDON, 1993)	HUMAN RESPONSE PATTERNS (FITZPATRICK, 1991)
	Value-Belief: Values, goals, or beliefs that guide choices or decisions.	**Relating:** To connect, to establish a link between, to stand in some association to another thing, person or place; to be borne or thrust in between things.
		Valuing: To be concerned about, to care; the worth or worthiness; the relative status of a thing, or the estimate in which it is held, according to its real or supposed worth, usefulness, or importance; one's opinion of liking for a person or thing; to equate in importance.

Remember:

- The better you are prepared for the interview, the better your chances of asking something revealing that provides new insights about the patient, which in turn will help you to ask more pertinent questions.

- The better listener you are, the better your chance of hearing something meaningful in the patient's responses.

- The more perceptive you are, the better your chances of seeing new relationships among the data collected.

take place over several contact sessions, but each contact should yield information, verify information already gathered, and/or clarify data. A well-conducted interview can be the first step in establishing a beneficial nurse-patient relationship and the rapport needed for good communication.

However, the interview is not merely the routine completion of the items on a standardized form by whomever is available. Rather, it is a tool of communication that permits an interactive exchange of information, a process that produces a higher level of understanding than that which either person could achieve alone. The nursing interview thus has a specific purpose: the collection of a set of specific data (information) from the patient and/or significant others through both conversation (subjective data) and observation (objective data). Box 2–1 provides some examples to clarify the distinction between these two forms of data.

Clearly the interview involves more than simply exchanging and processing data. Nonverbal communication is as important as the patient's choice of words in providing the data. The ability to collect data that is meaningful to the patient's health concerns depends heavily on your own knowledge base; the choice and sequence of questions; and the ability to give meaning to the patient's responses, integrate the data gathered, and prioritize the resulting information. Your knowledge, understanding, and insight into the nature and behavior of the patient are essential elements, as well.

Now take a few moments to read through Box 2–2, which identifies 10 key elements for a successful interview. As you begin to understand and apply these patient interviewing techniques, you will see that they provide an opportunity for the patient to use descriptive terms and to explain more fully

BOX 2-1 SUBJECTIVE DATA COMPARED WITH OBJECTIVE DATA

Subjective data are what the patient/significant other(s) say reflecting their own thoughts, feelings, and perceptions:

"My hip hurts." "I can't walk that far."
"I'm worried about surgery." "I don't know what to do."
"She didn't sleep well." "His usual weight is 160
"I can't give my husband a shot."   pounds."
"I haven't had a bowel movement "I don't think I'll ever get better."
  for 3 days."

Objective data are observable and measurable and include information gathered during the physical assessment and diagnostic studies:

Restless/agitated Cardiac murmur
Temperature 99.2°F Putrid odor
Old surgical scar Bloody vomitus
Flabby muscle tone Facial grimacing
Hgb 12.4 Glucose 107

BOX 2-2 ELEMENTS OF A SUCCESSFUL INTERVIEW

A successful interview has 10 key elements: (1) a clear sense of the underlying purpose for conducting the interview, (2) preliminary or background research before the interview begins, (3) a formal request of the interviewee to conduct the interview, (4) sound interviewing strategy, (5) effective use of icebreakers, (6) smoothly addressing the business of the interview, (7) good rapport between nurse and patient, (8) sensitivity to the patient's needs during the interview process, (9) adequate time for recovery following discussion of sensitive areas, and (10) closure.

1. **Underlying purpose:** The information gathered during the interview will be used in formulating the plan of care. Knowing the underlying purpose provides guidance in asking as well as answering questions, especially when areas that appear to be unrelated to the current situation may need to be pursued.

2. **Preliminary research:** Investigate the patient's and the family's current and previous situation. You can use resources such as records from the doctor's office, receiving department (e.g., emergency department) or prior admissions, as well as other health-team members. Make notes to identify key points because research often generates questions that should be written down so they are not lost. This preparation will assist you when formulating questions in the interview. The end result of the interview depends on what is put into it.

3. **Request to conduct the interview:** Formally requesting the interview is courteous and can clearly promote a positive interaction. Identify yourself to the patient and explain precisely the purpose of collecting the data and how that data will be used. Together, set a time for the

(Continued)

BOX 2–2   ELEMENTS OF A SUCCESSFUL INTERVIEW (Continued)

interview, giving consideration to the needs and severity of the patient's condition and the availability of significant others. Allow yourself as much time as possible to prepare. Your approach and attitude are important in helping the patient to be comfortable and to understand the importance of the interview. "Mr. Jones, I would like to ask you some questions about yourself and your illness, so that together we may plan your care," is a more positive approach than, "I need to know your history." The first approach not only sells the interview but stimulates the patient's thinking. The result is a more productive interview.

4. **Interview strategy:** Cover the details of the interview in accordance with the definition of its purpose with the patient. Preparation and planning give a sense of security and a plan to fall back on if things go slowly or unexpectedly wrong. This also allows a comfortable departure from the plan when conversation takes an unexplored path into productive channels. A new twist and a refreshing insight are the gold nuggets of interviewing, leading to information that otherwise might not have been remembered or shared.

5. **Icebreakers:** Icebreakers are the words and phrases that can put the patient at ease, set the stage, and promote a relaxed situation. They are the first bond of human communication and trust in this new relationship. How the icebreakers are used during the first few minutes may determine how and if the interview proceeds as the participants will make important decisions concerning the future of this relationship. The patient and/or significant others are making judgments about you, (that you are sincere, trustworthy, sensitive, professionally competent, or not).

   Some examples of icebreakers that might be used are the acknowledgement of what you know and see: "You've been admitted for surgery." A comment about the weather may also put the patient at ease. Offering something to drink, if allowed, and asking the patient how he or she prefers to be addressed also serves to promote an atmosphere of relaxation. When you sit down and appear relaxed and interested, this goal is more readily achieved.

6. **Business:** Get to the business at hand. Ask your prepared questions, using terminology the patient understands. Listen for answers and clues that will lead to other questions that you may not have anticipated. The relaxed informality that you have achieved needs to continue through this phase. Do not expect insights immediately; they usually come with time, increased comfort level, and trust.

7. **Rapport:** Call the participants by name, and monitor reactions to questions. Be careful not to bore or intimidate them with embarrassing questions. It is important to know when to shift gears, speed up, or slow down; or when to ask more challenging questions. Do not hurry the interview, and maintain eye contact as appropriate based on cultural belief systems.

(Continued)

BOX 2–2   ELEMENTS OF A SUCCESSFUL INTERVIEW (Continued)

8. **Sensitivity:** It may be necessary to ask questions about issues that involve sensitive areas for the patient. For example, questions about sexuality, lifestyle, or behaviors put the person at risk for sexually transmitted diseases (STDs, including human immunodeficiency virus/acquired immunodeficiency syndrome [HIV/AIDS]) may be perceived as threatening. The nurse needs to proceed gently toward these sensitive areas. Be alert to verbal/nonverbal cues that may indicate that the area of discussion is particularly sensitive for the individual. Ceasing exploration at this point demonstrates respect for the individual's rights/privacy and can enhance the trust between participants.

9. **Recovery:** Recover the rapport. If the sensitive areas have been approached slowly, the recovery period should be fairly easy to accomplish. Warmth and caring evidenced by a smile and the touch of the hand are helpful.

10. **Closure:** Conclude the interview by summarizing the highlights of the interview and leave the door open for further communication by asking the patient if he or she has anything else to add or any questions to ask of you.

---

the meaning of an answer. You will want to keep these tips in mind as you complete the practice activities in this chapter.

The interview question is the major tool you will use to obtain information. Box 2–3 lists nine effective data collection questioning techniques. How you phrase the question is a skill that is important in obtaining the desired results and getting the information necessary to make accurate nursing diagnoses. However, be aware that even with a properly phrased question, there will be times when the answer you are seeking will not be given. It is important to remember, too, that the patient has the right to refuse to answer any question at all, no matter how reasonably phrased. Box 2–4 highlights some questioning strategies to be avoided as they are generally ineffective in eliciting information from patients. At this point, take a moment to complete Practice Activity 2–1.

THE NURSING INTERVIEW: QUESTIONING AND LISTENING

The patient's MEDICAL DIAGNOSIS can provide a starting point for the nursing interview. Your knowledge about the anatomy and physiology of the disease/condition helps in choosing and prioritizing questions. Remember, though, that when using a nursing model assessment tool, the results of the focused interview will point to the human responses to health problems and to the development of nursing (rather than medical) diagnoses. Let us visit our first patient, Robert. Although you will ask Robert about the signs and symptoms associated with his pneumonia, your nursing focus will be:

- How does his shortness of breath affect his ability to care for himself? (Hygiene)

BOX 2–3   EFFECTIVE DATA COLLECTION TECHNIQUES

- **Open-ended questions** allow maximum freedom for the patient to respond in his or her own way; impose no limitations on how the question may be answered; and can produce considerable information, such as, "How do you feel about your new medications?" or "Explain the injection technique to me."
- **Hypothetical questions** pose a situation and ask the patient how it might be handled. You can learn whether the patient has accurate information and can think about how a similar situation might be handled. For example, "What would you do if you felt dizzy?" These questions may be very useful in determining the extent to which the patient has learned previously presented material.
- **Reflecting or "mirroring"** responses are useful techniques in getting at underlying meanings that might not be verbalized clearly. The patient might say, "Some days I'd like to throw this needle out the window." A mirror response might be, "You feel angry about the needle?" Now the patient is encouraged to verbalize what she or he is actually angry about. This response is nonevaluative and nonthreatening.
- **Focusing** shows the patient that you are attending to what is being said and consists of eye contact (within cultural limits), body posture, and verbal responses, that is, "Tell me more about that."
- **Giving broad openings** encourages the patient to take the initiative about what is to be talked about: "Where would you like to begin?"
- **Offering general leads** encourages the patient to continue: ". . . and then?"
- **Exploring** pursues a topic in more detail: "Would you describe it more fully."
- **Verbalizing the implied** gives voice to what has been suggested; for instance, the patient says, "It's no use taking this medicine anymore." You respond, "You're concerned that it isn't making a difference for you?"
- **Encouraging evaluation** helps the patient to consider the quality of his or her own experience, such as: "How does that seem to you?"

- Have the coughing episodes resulted in chest-wall pain or loss of sleep? (Pain/Discomfort, Activity/Rest)
- Has his appetite been affected by his frequent expectoration of purulent mucus? (Food/Fluid)
- How does he protect others from transmission of infection? (Safety, Teaching/Learning)

In addition, you need to keep an open mind and pay attention to clues that may identify other areas requiring investigation.

The Patient History

The history is more than simply recording information. You must review the data, organize and determine the relevance of each item (value the data), and document the facts. The quality of a history improves with your knowledge

---

BOX 2-4   GENERALLY INEFFECTIVE DATA COLLECTION TECHNIQUES

- **Closed-ended questions** (such as "Why?") allow little or no freedom in choosing a response, such as, "Do you take your medicine?" (patient responds "No") or "How long have you been taking insulin?" (patient responds "3 years"). Typically there are only one or two possible answers to the question. The interviewer remains in close control over the interview because of the rigid structure. Although the closed-ended question may be useful in an emergency situation (when it is necessary to gather information in a short time), it is important to provide an opportunity for asking the patient to explain the answers to these questions in greater detail.
- **Leading questions** typically suggest the desired response, such as, "The infection seems to be getting better, don't you agree?" and thereby reduce the range of responses because the interviewee most commonly agrees with any leading statement. Highly emotional questions, tone of voice, or inflection ("Where did you learn that injection technique?") may be heard as challenging, provoking the interviewee to "attack" or become defensive, thereby blocking communication.
- **Probing** is a persistent questioning, a demand for more information than is given willingly. "Now tell me about. . . ." This creates an uneasy feeling in the patient and may be interpreted as an invasion of privacy, resulting in a defensive response or withholding of information.
- **Agreeing/disagreeing** implies that the patient is "right" or "wrong" rather than promoting the patient's idea as separate from your own. This can block exploration of an issue. "I agree, that would be the thing to do," or "You didn't mean to do that, did you?"

---

and experience with the history-taking process. Although such assessments are often lengthy and time-consuming in the beginning, more time is eventually saved by avoiding the necessity to retrace steps, correct misinformation, and undo actions. With practice, the time required for this activity will decrease.

Guidelines for History-Taking

LISTEN CAREFULLY

Be a good listener: You need to listen attentively to what the individual is saying. Listen for whole thoughts and ideas, not merely isolated facts. Facts may not be as important as the ideas that bind them together. For example, Robert tells you, "Sure, my doctor ordered some pills for me [antibiotics for pneumonia], last month." But Robert's tone of voice, facial expression, and body language communicate the idea that he may not be following his treatment regimen. Robert's nonverbal communication requires validation by asking either reflecting or open-ended questions as described in Box 2–3. For example, "You seem to have a lack of enthusiasm as you tell me about your medication. What is that about?"

PRACTICE ACTIVITY 2–1

DETERMINING TYPES OF DATA

1. Identify Subjective (S) versus Objective (O) data:

_____ Skin cool/damp
_____ Sputum pale yellow
_____ Allergic to eggs and sulfa
_____ Pitting edema of feet and ankles
_____ Usually voids three times per day
_____ Chest pain lasting 15 minutes

2. Match the technique in column A to the statements in column B:

Column A	Column B
a. Open-ended question	_____ The next time this comes up, what would you do to handle it?
b. Hypothetical question	_____ That feeling in your chest, can you describe it more fully?
c. Reflection	_____ Do you use alcohol regularly?
d. Closed-ended question	_____ What would you like to talk about?
e. Leading question	_____ You're feeling better today, aren't you?

3. Rewrite the following using effective data collection techniques (see Box 2–3):

a. You felt like crying, didn't you? _____

b. You're in pain again? _____

c. Do you want to change occupations? _____

d. Since your doctor has talked with you, you don't have any questions, do you? _____

_____

e. Did you eat lunch? _____

ACTIVE LISTENING—
reflecting back what
the other person has
said to validate your
understanding of the
meaning. A restate-
ment of the other
person's total
communication,
including the words
and the feelings.

ACTIVE LISTENING

Use skills of active listening, silence, and acceptance to provide ample time for the person to respond: Give your full attention to the interview and do not interrupt. Save your own comments until the speaker is completely finished. Finally, ask related questions to stimulate the individual's memory if blocks occur. Once again, "facts" may not be as important as the patient's perception of reality. As you gain more experience in professional practice, you will begin to understand how important the patient's perception is. This will be especially true in your assessment, understanding, management, and treatment of your patient's reported perception of pain.

OBJECTIVITY

Be as objective as possible: Identify only the patient's and/or significant others' contributions to the history, and do not try to interpret the data at this point. Record subjective data from the patient/significant others just as it was stated during the interview. Failure to do so may cause confusion and lead to inaccurate diagnoses. However, lengthy responses may need to be paraphrased.

Your initial responsibility is to observe, collect, and record data without drawing conclusions or making judgments/assumptions. Your self-awareness is a crucial factor in the interaction, because perceptions, judgments, and assumptions can easily color the assessment findings unless they are recognized. We all have a responsibility to understand how our biases affect the conclusions we draw from the data and not be influenced by them. It may be useful to review the beliefs cited in Chapter 1 and the Code for Nurses contained in Appendix D.

MANAGEABLE DETAIL

Keep the amount of detail manageable: The data collected about the patient and/or significant others contain a vast amount of information, some of which may be repetitious. However, some of it will be valuable for eliciting information that was not recalled or volunteered previously.

Enough material needs to be noted in the history so that a complete picture is presented, and yet not so much that the information will not be read or used. "Necessary" information includes all data (positive and negative) that are relevant to the situation. For example, let us return to your patient Robert. He was admitted with the diagnosis of pneumonia. During the history he reports, "I've been coughing a lot lately." Necessary information in this case would be to clarify what Robert means by "coughing a lot lately." You need to know the frequency and time of coughing and factors that bring about or terminate an episode of coughing. Along with the cough you would want the necessary information about whether or not the cough was productive. So you would want to know the descriptive characteristics of the mucus. What color was it? How much mucus does he expectorate? As you can see, the "necessary" information is that information that will clarify and make the communication of Robert's subjective data to other healthcare providers both useful and meaningful.

SEQUENCE INFORMATION

Order is imperative: Develop and use a form that makes it easy to find information, identify problems, and choose nursing diagnoses. In addition, present the current health problems in chronologic order and include relevant events from the past. It is also useful to express topics in a uniform manner. For example, expressing the age at which events/illnesses/surgery occurred instead of just the year events occurred: "age 67/born 1923"; or "hysterectomy, age 35/1968."

DOCUMENT CLEARLY

Write legibly: This required skill improves the communication and comprehension of your findings, decreasing the chance of misunderstanding, saving time for you as well as other healthcare professionals who rely on your records.

RECORD DATA IN A TIMELY WAY

Write the history as soon as possible after gathering the information: This helps ensure greater accuracy of the data. The longer you wait to record, the more likely it is the data and specific details will fade and be more difficult to recall. A word of advice, data not written are data lost.

PHYSICAL EXAMINATION: THE HANDS-ON PHASE

You perform the physical examination to gather objective information, and also as a screening device. For the data collected during the physical examination to be meaningful, you need to know the normal physical and emotional characteristics of human beings sufficiently well enough to be able to recognize deviations.

Focus and Preparation

In order to gain as much information as possible from the assessment procedure, approach the patient with a positive, sincere attitude. Such an attitude conveys competence, interest, kindness, thoroughness, orderliness, and confidence. It may be frightening for the patient if you give the impression that you do not know what you are doing, or if you are awkward in performing assessment tasks. Give the patient a clear explanation of the procedures you will be using. Then, proceed with the examination according to the format you have previously chosen to gather and record the data: a nursing model (as suggested earlier), a systems approach (cardiovascular, respiratory, gastrointestinal, and so on), a head-to-toe approach (head, neck, chest, and so on), or a combination of these. The same format should be used each time you perform a physical examination to lessen the possibility of omissions and to increase your confidence and efficiency in completing the task.

However, the patient's state of health/severity of condition may require you to place priority on specific portions of your assessment. This priority in data collection is based in part on the measurement criteria developed by the ANA. "The priority of data collection is determined by the client's immediate condition or needs" (ANA, 1991). For example, when examining a patient with severe chest pain, you would probably choose to evaluate the pain and the cardiovascular system before addressing other areas. Likewise, the duration and length of any physical examination depends on circumstances such as the condition of the patient and the urgency of the situation.

During the examination, emotional support and care should be offered as indicated. Your professional judgment needs to be used in selecting the steps and sequencing the assessment to provide emotional support as needed. The patient with resolving chest pain may want to talk about his embarrassment of being perceived as "weak" during the episode of chest pain. Stopping your examination to support and listen to your patient is not only a correct intervention, but also demonstrates the sensitive blending of the art and science of nursing.

It is also important to provide the patient with as much feedback as possible. While completing the examination process, you will find this is an excellent opportunity to provide education on associated procedures, assessment findings, and health teaching in general. Perceptual and observational skills are especially important in determining what your patient needs.

Assessment Methods

Four common methods used during the physical examination are inspection, palpation, percussion, and auscultation. These techniques incorporate the senses of sight, hearing, touch, and smell:

1. *Inspection* is a systematic process of observation that is not limited to vision but also includes the senses of hearing and smell.

   Sight: Observing the skin for color, discolorations, lacerations; the lesion for drainage; the respiratory pattern for depth and symmetry; body language, movement, and posture, use of extremities, presence of physical limitations; the face for expressions, and so on.

   Hearing: Listening to the nature of a cough; the integrity of a joint; the tone of a voice or content of interactions with others, and so on.

   Smell: Detecting significant odors.

2. *Palpation* is the touching or pressing of the external surface of the body with the fingers.

   Touch: Feeling a lump; noting temperature, degree of moistness, and texture of skin; or determining strength of uterine contraction.

   Pressure: Determining the character of a pulse, evaluating edema, noting position of the fetus, or pinching (tenting) to observe skin turgor.

   Probing deeper: Reveals muscle tone/tension, or an abnormal pain response.

3. *Percussion* is the direct or indirect tapping of a specific body surface to ascertain information about underlying tissues or organs.

   Using fingertips: Tap the chest and listen for the sound indicating the presence or absence of fluid, masses, or consolidation.

   Using a percussion hammer: Tap the knee and observe the presence or absence of lower leg movement/reflexes.

4. *Auscultation* is listening for sounds within the body with the aid of a stethoscope and describing or interpreting them.

   Hearing: Listening at the antecubital space for blood pressure, the chest for heart/lung sounds, the abdomen for bowel sounds or fetal heart tones.

Follow-up Considerations

After completion of the physical examination, your patient may require assistance. The patient may need to be helped down off the examination table for safety reasons or may require help with dressing. Consideration of these sometimes forgotten needs enhances the rapport and trust developed during the examination. Including these interventions personalizes the patient-nurse interaction and makes the assessment process much more than just your hasty gathering of required data.

You may need to verify or clarify communication associated with the physical examination. By repeating aloud what you have observed, you give the patient the opportunity to validate the accuracy of the information obtained and misunderstandings can be avoided. For example, Observation: "I noticed that you flinched when I palpated your abdomen"; Response: "Yes your hand was cold and I'm ticklish."

LABORATORY AND DIAGNOSTIC STUDIES: SUPPORTING EVIDENCE

Laboratory and diagnostic studies are a part of the information-gathering stage. They aid in the management, maintenance, and restoration of health. Some tests are used to diagnose disease, whereas others are useful in following the course of a disease or adjusting therapy. Your knowledge about the purpose, procedure, and results of various scans, x-rays, performance tests (e.g., treadmill electrocardiogram, pulmonary function) and numerous laboratory studies is necessary both for the success of the study and to promote timely nursing intervention and a positive patient outcome through preparing and educating the patient about the prescribed studies.

In reviewing and interpreting laboratory tests, it is important to remember that the origin of the test material does not always correlate to an organ or body system. For example, a urine test might be done to detect the presence of bilirubin and urobilinogen, which could indicate liver disease, biliary obstruction, or hemolytic disease. In some cases, the relationship of the test to the pathology is clear, whereas in others, like obtaining renal function studies in the presence of cardiac failure, it is not. This is a result of the interrelationships between the various organs and systems of the body. In a few cases the results of a test are nonspecific, because they only indicate a disorder or abnormality and do not indicate where the cause of the problem is located. For example, an elevated sedimentation rate (ESR) suggests the presence but not the location of an inflammatory process.

In evaluating laboratory tests, it is advisable to consider which drugs are being administered to the patient, because these may have the potential to blur or falsify results, creating a misleading diagnostic picture.

For example:
- Heparin will prolong blood clotting times.
- Oral iron preparations cause a false-positive result when the stool is tested for occult blood.
- Phenazopyridine (Pyridium) is a urinary tract analgesic that can color the urine red.
- Use of promethazine (Phenergan), an antiemetic, can cause a false-negative result in a pregnancy test.

In some cases, it is necessary to note at what time medication was administered. Serum levels can be drawn to determine the varied concentrations of administered medications. Terms such as *peak* and *trough* levels are used to determine both the possible toxic effects and the therapeutic ranges of the medication.

There are also several mechanisms that may alter the laboratory results through the introduction of interfering materials.

For example:

- Food that gives a yellow color to blood serum (e.g., carrots, yams) will alter a bilirubin test.

- Food may contribute to the presence of substances in body fluids/excretions, such as hemoglobin and myoglobin in meat, which may lead to a misdiagnosis of occult blood in the stool.

- Intramuscular injections can elevate creatine phosphokinase (CPK) levels used to diagnose acute myocardial infarction.

ORGANIZING INFORMATION ELEMENTS

Clustering the Collected Data

Data gathered in the interview, in the physical examination, and from other records/sources, are organized and recorded in a concise systematic way and clustered into similar categories. Various formats have been used to accomplish this, including a review of body systems. The body systems approach has been used by both medicine and nursing for many years but is actually more useful for the physician in making a medical diagnosis than for a nurse in identifying nursing diagnoses. Currently nursing is developing and fine-tuning its own tools for recording and clustering data (e.g., Doenges & Moorhouse, 1993; Gordon, 1993; Guzzetta, et al., 1989). Organizing data using a nursing framework (Box 2–5) will assist you in focusing your attention and in choosing specific nursing diagnosis labels to describe the data accurately. However, it is important to be aware of the advantages of each type of framework, and to follow the approach recommended by your school or agency. Remember, consistency is the key. Before you complete Practice Activity 2–2, it is suggested you read the information in Box 2–6 and return to Table 2–1 to review the definitions of the 13 diagnostic divisions and the 11 functional health patterns.

Reviewing and Validating Findings

VALIDATION is an ongoing process that occurs during the data collection phase and on its completion, when the data are reviewed and compared. You review the data to be sure that what has been recorded is factual and to identify errors of omission or inconsistencies that require additional investigation. Validation is particularly important when the data are conflicting, when the source of the data may not be reliable, or when serious harm to the patient could result from any inaccuracies. Ask questions of the patient or others to

VALIDATION—
the process of assuring that data are factual.

BOX 2–5   ASSESSMENT DATA AND APPLICATION TO EXCERPT FROM DOENGES AND MOORHOUSE DIAGNOSTIC DIVISIONS ASSESSMENT TOOL

Respiration

REPORTS (SUBJECTIVE)

Dyspnea, related to: Climbing stairs/walking more than two blocks, close places/crowds
   Cough/sputum: Thick, yellow, approximately 1/4 tsp, 6 to 10 times/day, especially with activity
History of:
   Bronchitis: Diagnosed 1987
   Asthma: No   *Tuberculosis:* No
   Emphysema: Diagnosed 1987
   Recurrent pneumonia: Yes; last admission approximately 6 months ago
   Exposure to noxious fumes: Not aware of past exposures (diesel trucker)
Smoker: Cigarettes (pack/day): 1×45 years, $1/2 \times 8$ years (since 1987)
   Number of pack/years: 49
Use of respiratory aids: Inhaler and PO meds
Oxygen: No/"Doctor suggested I use oxygen at night, but I don't think I'm that bad."

EXHIBITS (OBJECTIVE)

Respiratory: Rate: 28 at rest   *Depth:* Shallow
   Symmetry: Increased AP diameter
Use of accessory muscles: Yes
Nasal flaring: None observed
Fremitus: Increased tactile   *Egophone:* Resonance increased
   Percussion: Hyperresonate
Breath sounds: Diminished, bronchovesicular, basilar inspiratory crackles bilateral, scattered rhonchi—limited clearing with cough
Cyanosis: Oral mucous membranes pale
Clubbing of fingers: Slight
Sputum characteristics: Yellow, tenacious, scant amount during assessment
Mentation/restlessness: Alert; responds to all questions; no restlessness
Other: Verbal responses slow; breathless—phrases 4 to 5 words long
Results chest x-ray: Bilateral lower lobe infiltrates

On reviewing the collected data for this patient with pneumonia and noting cues (signs and symptoms) in the Respiration section of the data base, you are referred to the Respiration section of the Diagnostic Divisions. Four possible labels are suggested: Airway Clearance, ineffective; Aspiration, risk for; Breathing Pattern, ineffective; and Gas Exchange, impaired.

PRACTICE ACTIVITY 2–2

ORGANIZING DATA: DIAGNOSTIC DIVISIONS AND FUNCTIONAL HEALTH PATTERNS

Donald has been admitted to the psychiatric hospital inpatient substance abuse unit for treatment of depression and withdrawal from alcohol.

Organize the data below according to diagnostic divisions and functional health patterns. Place the number of the listed data next to the category where you believe it fits (see Table 2–1).

1. 46-year-old male
2. Divorced, not currently involved in a relationship
3. Loan banker, laid off 7 months ago.
4. Unsteady gait
5. Clothes rumped, has not shaved for 2 days, dry skin
6. Eats 1 or 2 meals a day—donuts, sandwiches, meat and potatoes, no vegetables or fruits; coffee 4+ cups/day
7. Stools have been loose, 3 to 4/day
8. BP 136/82 (right arm/sitting), radial pulse 92
9. Alert and oriented
10. Catholic, not practicing
11. Sleeps usually 3 to 4 hours a night, awakens around 5:00 AM
12. "I've been drinking a lot lately." Bourbon 1 fifth/day
13. Worries about financial situation, unable to make support payments
14. Congested nonproductive cough
15. Reports constant throbbing pain, left knee—old sports injury
16. Genogram:

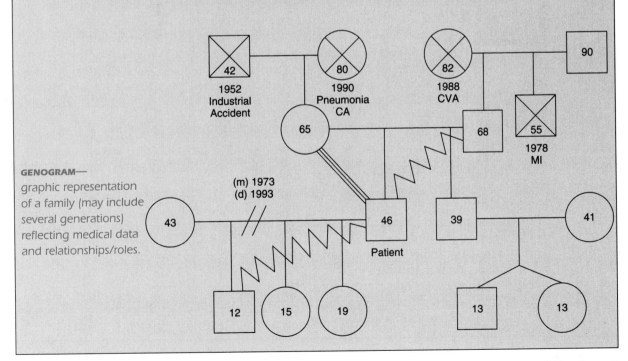

GENOGRAM—
graphic representation of a family (may include several generations) reflecting medical data and relationships/roles.

(Continued)

PRACTICE ACTIVITY 2–2 (Continued)

Diagnostic Divisions

Activity/Rest:
Circulation:
Ego Integrity:
Elimination:
Food/Fluid:
Hygiene:
Neurosensory:
Pain/Discomfort:
Respiration:
Safety:
Sexuality:
Social Interaction:
Teaching/Learning:

Functional Health Patterns

Health Perception/Health Management:
Nutritional/Metabolic:
Elimination:
Activity/Exercise:
Cognitive/Perceptual:
Sleep/Rest:
Self-Perception/Self-Concept:
Role/Relationship:
Sexuality/Reproductive:
Coping/Stress Tolerance:
Value/Belief:

BOX 2–6   ORGANIZING ASSESSMENT DATA USING A NURSING FRAMEWORK

The following data is information you obtained for the patient data base during your assessment of Michelle (following her admission to the orthopedic unit having had an external fixation device applied for multiple compound fractures of the right lower leg). The data have been clustered in each of three nursing frameworks by means of the identifying numbers for each data element.

Assessment Data

1. 14-year-old female
2. High-school student
3. Practicing Baptist
4. Single
5. Living with parents, one older brother, one younger sister
6. Temperature 100°F
7. Sharp severe pain, right lower leg, "toes to knees," rated "9" on 0 to 10 scale, and rightsided headache rated "4."
8. Hospitalized for tonsillectomy 4 years ago
9. Alert and oriented, brief loss of consciousness at time of injury
10. Respirations 26, lungs clear, splinting with deep inspiration
11. Weight 98 pounds
12. Indwelling catheter in place, urine clear, amber
13. Independent in self-care
14. Usually sleeps 8 hours each night
15. Right lower leg—wound packed with sterile dressing; multiple puncture sites (external fixator in place)
16. Menarche at age 13

(Continued)

BOX 2-6 ORGANIZING ASSESSMENT DATA USING A NURSING FRAMEWORK (Continued)

17. Manages stress by talking with friends, exercise (distance runner and mountain biking)
18. States has no allergies
19. Concerned that injury will leave scars and affect participation in track activities
20. P 110, BP 100/78 (left arm/supine)

How you organize this data is dependent on the format you choose for recording. On occasion, data may be recorded in more than one section as the divisions/patterns are based on human responses instead of specific body systems. The above data could be recorded in three different nursing formats, thus:

Doenges and Moorhouse: Diagnostic Divisions

Activity/Rest: 2, 9, 14, 17
Circulation: 20
Ego integrity: 3, 4, 17, 19
Elimination: 12
Food/Fluid: 11
Hygiene: 13
Neurosensory: 9

Pain/Discomfort: 7
Respiration: 10
Safety: 6, 15, 18
Sexuality: 1, 4, 16
Social interaction: 4, 5
Teaching/Learning: 2, 8

Gordon's: Functional Health Patterns

Health Perception/Health
    Management: 7, 8
Nutritional/Metabolic: 6, 10, 11,
    15, 18, 20
Coping/Stress Tolerance: 17
Value/Belief: 3
Cognitive/Perceptual: 9

Self-perception/Self-concept: 19
Role/Relationship: 1, 2, 4, 5
Sexuality/Reproductive: 4, 16
Elimination: 12
Activity/Exercise: 10, 13, 17
Sleep/Rest: 14

NANDA: Human Response Patterns

Exchanging: 6, 8, 10, 11, 12, 15,
    18, 20
Communicating: 0
Relating: 1, 2, 4, 5, 16
Valuing: 3

Moving: 13, 14
Perceiving: 19
Knowing: 9
Feeling: 7
Choosing: 17

verify your impressions; for example, "Tell me more about that." "What I heard you say is. . . ." Validating the information gathered can avoid the possibility of making wrong inferences or conclusions that can lead to inaccurate nursing diagnoses, incorrect outcomes, and/or inappropriate nursing actions. This can be done by sharing your assumptions with the individuals involved and having them verify the accuracy of those conclusions.

BOX 2–7   MEASUREMENT CRITERIA FOR ANA STANDARD I

Assessment: The nurse collects client health data.

1. The priority of data collection is determined by the client's immediate condition or needs.
2. Pertinent data are collected using appropriate assessment techniques.
3. Data collection involves client, significant others, and healthcare providers when appropriate.
4. The data collection process is systematic and ongoing.
5. Relevant data are documented in a retrievable form.

Data that are grossly abnormal are rechecked, and objective and subjective data are compared for congruencies and/or inconsistencies. For example, the patient reports upper right abdominal pain, although musculature appears relaxed and the patient does not flinch on abdominal palpation. Additional investigation reveals that the pain is episodic and usually follows meal times. Temporary factors that may affect the data are also identified/noted. For example, you note the patient's right hand is cool in comparison with the left hand. On questioning her, you discover she had been holding a glass of ice water in her right hand.

Finally, the patient may remember something, or feel more comfortable in sharing information with you, and although the data collected by any healthcare professional are confidential, it may be appropriate or necessary to share the information. For example, you may have a greater opportunity to observe interactions between family members during the assessment process that could have an impact on the diagnostic process and/or the plan of care. Some of these findings may need to be brought to the attention of other healthcare professionals, such as the physician, dietician, or physical therapist. Sharing this additional data aids in collaborative planning of care.

SUMMARY

The assessment step of the nursing process emphasizes and should provide a holistic view of the patient. The generalized assessment done during the overall gathering of data creates a profile of the patient. A focused assessment may be done to obtain more information about a specific issue that needs expansion or clarification. Both types of assessment are important, and complement each other. A successfully completed assessment will provide data on the patient's state of wellness, response to health problems, and risk factors.

Now, before we briefly describe the next chapter, let us return to the first ANA Standard of Clinical Nursing Practice and review the measurement criteria necessary to achieve and ensure compliance with the standard. The knowledge and skill required to meet the criteria listed in Box 2–7 have been described in this chapter.

The next chapter presents the second step of the nursing process—Problem Identification. In this upcoming chapter, the diagnostic reasoning process will be used to analyze/synthesize the information obtained from the patient data base, and identify the patient healthcare needs or nursing diagnoses that form the basis for the development of the plan of care.

WORK PAGE: Chapter Two

1. Rewrite the following questions so that they are open-ended:

   a. You're feeling better after the respiratory treatment, aren't you? _____

   _____

   b. Have you taken your medicine today? _____

   _____

   c. Do you understand these directions? _____

   _____

2. Using the technique of reflection, write a question to clarify these patient statements:

   a. Do you think I should tell my doctor about my concern? _____

   _____

   b. What do you want to talk about today? _____

   _____

   c. I don't think I can go on without my husband. _____

   _____

   d. Do you think it is important to get married? _____

   _____

3. When might a closed-ended question be helpful?

   _____

4. Describe the three components of the patient data base:

   a. _____   b. _____   c. _____

5. The four activities involved in the physical assessment are:

   a. _____   b. _____   c. _____   d. _____

6. The patient data base is important to the provision of patient care because

   _____

7. For assessment purposes the difference between subjective data and objective data is _____

_____

_____

8. Underline the subjective data, and circle the objective data in the following vignette:

Vignette: Sally comes to the obstetric department for evaluation of her stage of labor. Back pains began about 3 hours ago (8 PM) while on her job as a respiratory therapist. Contractions are 5 minutes apart, lasting 30 seconds for the last 45 minutes. BP 146/84 (left arm/lying), P 110, respirations 24. Weight 155 pounds (up 4 pounds this week). Cervix dilated 4 cm, membranes intact. Fetal head engaged, heart tones slightly muffled in right lower quadrant, rate 132. Nauseated since a dinner of fried chicken 4 hours ago. Appears anxious and seems irritated that her physician is not here. Voided 1 hour ago, has not had a bowel movement for 2 days. Stopped smoking 8 months ago. Lungs clear. No allergies. Married, husband plans to attend the birth. Two children are in the care of their grandmother tonight. Appearance is well-groomed with a well-fitting maternity uniform and low-heeled shoes. Requests to leave contacts in to observe the birth. Last physical examination 1 week ago. Gestation 37 weeks, with due date 3 weeks off—3/11/95.

9. An important benefit of doing "research" or reviewing available information before an interview

is _____

_____

10. An interview should be "requested" because _____

_____

11. Check those information resources that can be useful in helping the nurse to prepare for the interview:

_____ Family/significant other   _____ Physician notes

_____ Old medical records   _____ Textbooks/reference journals

_____ Diagnostic studies   _____ Other nurses/healthcare providers

12. Sensitivity of the nurse is important during the interview process to _____

_____

13. List three abilities of the nurse that are necessary in order to collect a relevant patient data base.

a. _____ b. _____ c. _____

14. In the following vignette, cluster and record the assessment data (following the numbers) into the appropriate diagnostic divisions listed below. Refer to Table 2–1 as needed for the type of data included in the specific divisions to assist you in clustering the data.

Vignette: Robert, a 72-year-old (1) male admitted to the medical unit at 1:00 PM for (2) bilateral lower lobe pneumonia. (3) Has had liquids only by mouth for several days. (4) Last BM—2 days ago, brown/formed stool, (5) voided at 1:20 PM—clear, dark amber. He reports (6) "My chest hurts", as he splints chest while coughing. (7) Small amount, thick, yellow sputum expectorated with cough. (8) Appears anxious, fidgeting with sheets, face tense, watching nurse intently. (9) Tympanic (TMT) temperature 101°F, (10) BP 178/102 (left arm/lying), P 100/regular, (11) respirations 28/shallow. (12) Skin warm, moist, color pale. (13) Has difficulty hearing questions, left hearing aid (R ear) at home. (14) Reports "This is the second episode in a month." (15) Doctor did prescribe antibiotic (drug unknown) a month ago, patient did not complete treatment. (16) States he lives alone (widower), and is (17) responsible for meeting his own needs. In reviewing diagnostic studies, you note the (18) chest x-ray reveals infiltrates both lower lobes and a (19) Gram stain of the sputum reveals gram-negative bacteria.

DIAGNOSTIC DIVISIONS

Activity/Rest: _____
Circulation: _____
Ego Integrity: _____
Social Interaction: _____
Respiration: _____
Food/Fluid: _____

Hygiene: _____
Neurosensory: _____
Pain/Discomfort: _____
Elimination: _____
Teaching/Learning: _____

Safety: _____
Sexuality: _____

BIBLIOGRAPHY

American Nurses' Association. (1980). *Nursing: A Social Policy Statement.* St. Louis, MO: Author.

American Nurses' Association. (1991). *Standards of Clinical Nursing Practice.* St. Louis, MO: Author.

Burley, J.T. (1993). *Instructor's Guide for Nursing Care Plans: Guidelines for Planning and Documenting Patient Care and Nurse's Pocket Guide: Nursing Diagnoses with Interventions.* Philadelphia: F.A. Davis.

Doenges, M.E., Moorhouse, M.E., & Geissler, A.C. (1993). *Nursing Care Plans: Guidelines for Planning and Documenting Patient Care* (3rd ed.). Philadelphia: F.A. Davis.

Fitzpatrick, J.J. (1991). In R.M. Carroll-Johnson (Ed.) *Classification of Nursing Diagnosis: Proceedings of the Ninth Conference.* Philadelphia: J.B. Lippincott.

Gordon, M. (1993). *Nursing Diagnosis: Process and Application* (3rd ed.). St. Louis, MO: C.V. Mosby.

Guzzetta, C.E., Bunton, S.D., Prinkey, L.A., Sherer, A.P., & Seifert, P.C. (1989). *Clinical Assessment Tools for Use with Nursing Diagnoses.* St. Louis, MO: C.V. Mosby.

SUGGESTED READING

Billings, J.A., & Stoeckle, J.D. (1989). *The Clinical Encounter: A Guide to the Medical Interview and Case Presentation.* Chicago: Year Book Medical.

Cohen-Cole, S.A. (1991). *The Medical Interview: The Three-Function Approach.* St. Louis, MO: Mosby–Year Book.

Coulehan, J.L., & Block, M.R. (1992). *The Medical Interview: A Primer for Students of the Art* (2nd ed.). Philadelphia: F.A. Davis.

Hogstel, M.O., & Keen-Payne, R. (1993). *Practical Guide to Health Assessment: Through the Lifespan.* Philadelphia: F.A. Davis.

Malasanos, L., Barkauskas, V., & Stoltenberg-Allen, K. (1990). *Health Assessment* (5th ed.). St. Louis, MO: C.V. Mosby.

Murray, R. (1989). *Nursing Assessment and Health Promotion Strategies Through the Life Span* (4th ed.). Norwalk, CT: Appleton & Lange.

Seidel, H.M., Ball, J.W., Dains, J.E., & Benedict, G.W. (1991). *Mosby's Guide to Physical Examination (2nd ed.).* St. Louis, MO: Mosby–Year Book.

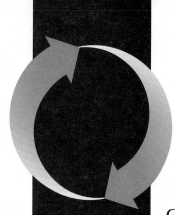

CHAPTER 3

The Problem Identification Step: Analyzing the Data

ANA Standard 2: *Diagnosis: The nurse analyzes the assessment data in determining diagnoses.*

The second step of the nursing process is often referred to as ANALYSIS, as well as PROBLEM IDENTIFICATION or NURSING DIAGNOSIS. Although all of these terms may be used interchangeably, the purpose of this step of the nursing process is to draw conclusions regarding a patient's specific problems or needs so that effective care can be planned and delivered. We have chosen to label this step of the nursing process *problem identification*. To be more specific, problem identification is a process of data analysis using diagnostic reasoning (a form of clinical judgment) in which judgments, decisions, and conclusions are made about the meaning of the data collected, in order to determine whether or not nursing intervention is indicated.

ANALYSIS—the process of examining and categorizing information to reach a conclusion about a patient's needs.

PROBLEM IDENTIFICATION—the second step of the nursing process, in which the data collected are analyzed and, through the process of diagnostic reasoning, specific patient diagnostic statements are created.

39

NURSING DIAGNOSIS
—**Noun:** a label approved by NANDA identifying specific patient problems/ needs. The means of describing health problems amenable to treatment by nurses; may be physical, sociological, or psychological.
—**Verb:** the process of identifying specific patient problems/ needs; used by some as the title of the second step of the nursing process.

DIAGNOSIS—Forming a clinical judgment identifying a disease/condition or human response through scientific evaluation of signs/symptoms, history, and diagnostic studies.

The DIAGNOSIS of patient problems has been done by nurses on an informal basis since the early beginnings of the profession. The term came into formal use in the nursing literature during the 1950s, although its meaning continued to be seen in the context of medical diagnosis. A group of interested nursing leaders met and held a national conference in 1973. Their purpose was to identify the patient problems that fall within the scope of nursing, label them, and develop a classification system that could be used by nurses throughout the world. This group called these labels *nursing diagnoses*. Regional, national, and international workshops and conferences continue to be held since the first conference. The North American Nursing Diagnosis Association (NANDA) meets every 2 years to review their work on the development and classification of nursing diagnoses, as well as the work of other nursing groups, representing various clinical specialties and healthcare settings.

American Nurses' Association (ANA) standards of practice were first developed in 1973, and with the acceptance of the ANA Social Policy Statement in 1980, which defined nursing as the "diagnosis and treatment of human responses to actual or potential health problems," the movement for broad use of a common language was enhanced. The system developed by NANDA meets this need. It provides a standard terminology that is accepted by ANA and various specialty groups and is being used across the United States and in many countries around the world. The NANDA list has also been proposed for inclusion in the World Health Organization's *International Classification of Diseases: Conditions that Necessitate Nursing Care*.

Today, the use of the nursing process and nursing diagnoses is rapidly becoming an integral part of an effective system of nursing practice. It is a system that can be used within existing conceptual frameworks, because it is a generic approach adaptable to all academic and clinical settings.

DEFINING NURSING DIAGNOSIS

The term *nursing diagnosis* has been used as both a verb and a noun. This may result in confusion. Nursing diagnosis is used as a noun in reference to the work of NANDA. For the purposes of this text, *nursing diagnosis* will refer to the NANDA list of nursing diagnosis labels (Table 3–1) that form the stem of the PATIENT DIAGNOSTIC STATEMENT.

PATIENT DIAGNOSTIC STATEMENT—the outcome of the diagnostic reasoning process; a three-part statement identifying the patient's problem/ need, the etiology of the problem/need, and the associated signs/ symptoms.

Although nurses work within the nursing, medical, and psychosocial domains, nursing's phenomena of concern are patterns of human response, *not* disease processes. Therefore, nursing diagnoses do not parallel medical/psychiatric diagnoses but *do* involve independent nursing activities as well as collaborative roles and actions.

The nursing diagnosis is a conclusion drawn from the data collected about a patient that serves as a means of describing a health problem amenable to treatment by nurses. A uniform or standardized way of identifying, focusing on, and labeling specific phenomena allows the nurse to deal effectively with individual patient responses.

Although there are different definitions of the term *nursing diagnosis*, NANDA has accepted the following working definition:

Nursing diagnosis is a clinical judgment about individual, family, or community responses to actual and potential health problems/life

Table 3-1 **NURSING DIAGNOSES**

Accepted for Use and Research (1995)

Activity Intolerance [specify level]
Activity Intolerance, risk for
Adaptive Capacity: Intracranial, decreased
Adjustment, impaired
Airway Clearance, ineffective
Anxiety [specify level]*
Aspiration, risk for

Body Image disturbance
Body Temperature, altered, risk for
Bowel Incontinence
Breastfeeding, effective
Breastfeeding, ineffective
Breastfeeding, interrupted
Breathing Pattern, ineffective

Cardiac Output, decreased
Caregiver Role Strain
Caregiver Role Strain, risk for
Communication, impaired, verbal
Community Coping, enhanced, potential for
Community Coping, ineffective
Confusion, acute
Confusion, chronic
Constipation
Constipation, colonic
Constipation, perceived
Coping, defensive
Coping, Individual, ineffective

Decisional Conflict (specify)
Denial, ineffective
Diarrhea
Disuse Syndrome, risk for
Diversional Activity deficit
Dysreflexia

Energy Field, disturbance
Environmental Interpretation Syndrome, impaired

Family Coping, ineffective: compromised
Family Coping, ineffective: disabling
Family Coping: potential for growth
Family Process, altered: Alcoholism
Family Processes, altered
Fatigue
Fear
Fluid Volume deficit [active loss]*
Fluid Volume deficit [regulatory failure]*
Fluid Volume deficit, risk for
Fluid Volume excess

Gas Exchange, impaired
Grieving, anticipatory
Grieving, dysfunctional
Growth and Development, altered

(Continued)

Table 3-1 NURSING DIAGNOSES (Continued)

Health Maintenance, altered
Health-Seeking Behaviors (specify)
Home Maintenance Management, impaired
Hopelessness
Hyperthermia
Hypothermia

Incontinence, functional
Incontinence, reflex
Incontinence, stress
Incontinence, total
Incontinence, urge
Infant Behavior, disorganized
Infant Behavior, disorganized, risk for
Infant Behavior, organized, potential for enhancement
Infant Feeding Pattern, ineffective
Infection, risk for
Injury, risk for

Knowledge deficit [Learning Need] (specify)*

Lonliness, risk for

Memory, impaired

Noncompliance, [Compliance, altered] specify*
Nutrition, altered, less than body requirements
Nutrition, altered, more than body requirements
Nutrition, altered, risk for more than body requirements

Oral Mucous Membrane, altered

Pain [acute]*
Pain, chronic
Parent/Infant/Child Attachment, altered, risk for
Parental Role conflict
Parenting, altered
Parenting, altered, risk for
Perioperative Positioning Injury, risk for
Peripheral Neurovascular dysfunction, risk for
Personal Identity disturbance
Physical Mobility, impaired
Poisoning, risk for
Post-Trauma Response
Powerlessness
Protection, altered
Rape-Trauma Syndrome
Rape-Trauma Syndrome: compound reaction
Rape-Trauma Syndrome: silent reaction
Relocation Stress Syndrome
Role Performance, altered

Self Care deficit (specify): feeding, bathing/hygiene, dressing/grooming, toileting
Self Esteem, chronic low
Self Esteem disturbance
Self Esteem, situational low
Self-Mutilation, risk for
Sensory/Perceptual alterations (specify): visual, auditory, kinesthetic, gustatory, tactile, olfactory
Sexual dysfunction
Sexuality Patterns, altered

(Continued)

Table 3–1   NURSING DIAGNOSES (Continued)

Skin Integrity, impaired
Skin Integrity, impaired, risk for
Sleep Pattern disturbance
Social Interaction, impaired
Social Isolation
Spiritual Distress (distress of the human spirit)
Spiritual Well Being, potential for enhancement
Spontaneous Ventilation, inability to sustain
Suffocation, risk for
Swallowing, impaired

Therapeutic Regimen: Community, ineffective management
Therapeutic Regimen: Families, ineffective management
Therapeutic Regimen: Individual, effective
Therapeutic Regimen: Individual, ineffective management
Thermoregulation, ineffective
Thought Processes, altered
Tissue Integrity, impaired
Tissue Perfusion, altered (specify): cerebral, cardiopulmonary, renal, gastrointestinal, peripheral
Trauma, risk for

Unilateral Neglect
Urinary Elimination, altered
Urinary Retention [acute/chronic]*

Ventilatory Weaning Response, dysfunctional (DVWR)
Violence, risk for, directed at self/others

*Information that appears in brackets has been added by the authors to clarify and facilitate the use of
 nursing diagnoses.

Distinguishing between Medical and Nursing Diagnoses. . . .

- **Medical Diagnoses** are illnesses/conditions, reflecting alteration of the structure or function of organs/systems, verified by medical diagnostic studies, such as diabetes, heart failure, hepatitis, cancer, and pneumonia. The medical diagnosis usually does not change.

- **Nursing Diagnoses** address human responses to actual and potential health problems/life processes, such as Activity Intolerance [specify level]; Health Maintenance, altered; Airway Clearance, ineffective; Self Care deficit (specify). The nursing diagnoses change as the patient's situation or perspective changes/resolves.

processes. Nursing diagnoses provide the basis for selection of nursing interventions to achieve outcomes for which the nurse is accountable.

The nursing diagnosis is as correct as the current data will allow because it is supported by that data. It says what the patient's situation is at the present time and reflects changes in the patient's condition as they occur. Each decision the nurse makes is time-dependent and, with additional information gathered later, decisions may change. Unlike medical diagnoses, nursing diagnoses change as the patient progresses through various stages of illness/maladaptation, to resolution of the problem or to the conclusion of the condition. For example, for a patient undergoing cardiac surgery, initial problems/needs may be Pain [acute]; Cardiac Output, decreased; Airway Clearance, ineffective; and Infection, risk for. As the patient progresses, problems/needs may shift to Activity Intolerance, risk for; Knowledge deficit [Learning Need] (specify); and Role Performance, altered.

THE USE OF NURSING DIAGNOSES

Although not yet comprehensive, the current NANDA list of diagnostic labels defines/refines professional nursing activity. The list of labels is now at a point where nurses need to use the proposed diagnoses on a daily basis, becoming familiar with the parameters of each individual diagnosis, and identifying its strengths and weaknesses, thus promoting research and further development.

The question is frequently asked: "Why should we use a nursing diagnosis . . . what is its value to the nursing profession?" There are many benefits that the use of a nursing diagnosis can provide. The accurate choice of a nursing diagnosis to label a patient problem/need:

- *Gives Nurses a Common Language:* Promotes improved communication among nurses, between shifts and units, other healthcare providers, and alternate care settings.

  For example: Using the nursing diagnosis "Airway Clearance, ineffective" instead of saying "difficulty breathing" conveys a distinct image. When hearing the former, a clear picture begins to develop in your mind, as your thoughts focus on the musculature of the upper airway, mucus production, and cough effort. With the second label, you do not have a clear idea as to what is happening with this patient, and you question whether the patient is experiencing a problem of maintaining an airway, movement of the chest, or perfusion to the lungs.

  This improved communication may result in improved quality and continuity of the care provided to the patient.

- *Promotes Identification of Appropriate Goals:* Aids in the choice of correct nursing interventions to alleviate the identified problem/need, and provides guidance for evaluation. Whereas nursing actions were once based on variables such as SIGNS and SYMPTOMS, test results, or a medical diagnosis, nursing diagnosis is a uniform way of identifying, focusing on, and dealing with specific patient responses to actual and potential health problems/needs (i.e., the phenomena of concern for nurses).

  For example: "Risk for infection" compared with "presence of urinary catheter." The high risk or potential threat of an infection brings to mind specific goals/outcomes and interventions to protect the patient, but what is your concern, if any, with the urinary catheter?

- *Provides Acuity Information:* Ranks the amount of work that requires nursing care and can serve as a basis for patient classification systems. This method of ranking can be used to determine individual staffing needs. It can also serve as documentation to provide justification for third-party reimbursement.

  For example: Nursing diagnoses can be given different, weighted values according to the degree of nursing involvement required; that is, "Gas Exchange, impaired," may require a considerable amount of skilled nursing time in order to promote adequate ventilation, to provide oxygen and respiratory treatments, and to monitor laboratory studies. "Acute Urinary Retention" may require a much shorter period of time to insert a catheter into the bladder and periodically measure the urine output.

  In addition, some third-party payors (such as Medicare and other insurance companies) include nursing diagnoses when considering extended length of stay or delayed discharge.

SIGN—objective or observable evidence or manifestation of a health problem.

SYMPTOM—subjectively perceptible change in the body or its functions that indicates disease or the kind or phases of disease.

- *Can Create a Standard for Nursing Practice:* Provides a foundation for quality assurance programs, a means of evaluating nursing practice, and a mechanism of costing-out delivery of nursing care.

  For example: Did the nursing interventions address and resolve the problem? Did the patient experience the desired result (for instance, alleviation of pain)? Were the goals met, or is there documentation of the reasons why they were not met? Were the expected outcomes changed to meet changing patient needs?

- *Provides a Quality Improvement Base:* Clinicians, administrators, educators, and researchers can document, validate, or alter the process of care delivery, which then improves the profession.

  For example: The use of universally understood labels enhances retrieval of specific data for review to determine accuracy, to validate and/or change nursing actions related to specific nursing diagnoses, and to evaluate an individual nurse's performance.

IDENTIFYING PATIENT PROBLEMS/NEEDS

During the Assessment step, the collection, clustering, and validation of patient data flow directly into the Problem Identification step of the nursing process, where you sense problems and choose nursing diagnoses.

Diagnostic Reasoning: Analyzing the Patient Data Base

Identifying patient problems/needs and then selecting a nursing diagnosis label involves the use of experience, expertise, and intuition on your part. There are six steps involved in problem identification that comprise the activities of diagnostic reasoning. The result is the creation of a patient diagnostic statement that identifies the patient problem, suggests its potential cause or etiology, and notes its signs and symptoms. This is known as the (P)roblem, (E)tiology, and (S)igns and symptoms, or P E S format (Gordon, 1976).

STEP 1: PROBLEM-SENSING

Data are reviewed and analyzed to identify CUES (signs and symptoms) suggesting patient problems or needs that can be described by nursing diagnosis labels. If the data have been recorded in a nursing format (e.g., Diagnostic Divisions, Functional Health Patterns, or Human Responses), the nurse is automatically guided to specific groups of nursing diagnoses when certain cues from the data are identified (Box 3–1). This helps to focus attention on appropriate diagnoses. Reviewing the NANDA definitions of specific diagnoses (see Appendix A) can be of further assistance in deciding between two or more similar diagnostic labels; for instance, there are five different diagnoses for urinary incontinence (see step 4).

  For example: When using the Diagnostic Divisions format, body temperature is recorded in the Safety section. When the patient temperature rises, the nurse reviews the diagnostic labels under Safety to find a possible fit, such as, *Hyperthermia* or *Infection, risk for.* At the same time, cues are noted in other sections of the data base that may be combined with fever

Remember . . . nursing diagnoses may be a physical, sociological, or psychological finding:

Physical Nursing Diagnoses include those which pertain to circulation (for example, Tissue Perfusion, altered [specify]), ventilation (for example, Airway Clearance, ineffective), elimination (for example, Constipation), and so on.

Psychosocial Nursing Diagnoses include those that pertain to the mind (for example, Thought Processes, altered), emotion (for example, Anxiety [specify level]), or lifestyle/relationships (for example, Sexuality Patterns, altered, or Social

CUE—a signal that indicates a possible need/direction for care.

BOX 3–1   *NURSING DIAGNOSES ORGANIZED ACCORDING TO DIAGNOSTIC DIVISIONS*

After data have been collected and areas of concern/need have been identified, consult the Diagnostic Divisions framework to review the list of nursing diagnoses that fall within the individual categories. This will assist with the choice of the specific diagnostic labels to accurately describe the data from the patient data base. Then, with the addition of etiology (when known) and signs and symptoms, the patient diagnostic statement emerges.

Diagnostic Division: Activity/Rest

Ability to engage in necessary/desired activities of life (work and leisure) and to obtain adequate sleep/rest

DIAGNOSES

Activity Intolerance [specify level]
Activity Intolerance, risk for
Disuse Syndrome, risk for
Diversional Activity deficit
Fatigue
Sleep Pattern disturbance

Diagnostic Divisions: Circulation

Ability to transport oxygen and nutrients necessary to meet cellular needs

DIAGNOSES

Adaptive Capacity: Intracranial, decreased
Cardiac Output, decreased
Dysreflexia
Tissue Perfusion, altered (specify): cerebral, cardiopulmonary, renal, gastrointestinal, peripheral

Diagnostic Division: Ego Integrity

Ability to develop and use skills and behaviors to integrate and manage life experiences

DIAGNOSES

Adjustment, impaired
Anxiety [specify level]
Body Image disturbance
Coping, defensive
Coping, Individual, ineffective
Decisional Conflict (specify)
Denial, ineffective
Energy Field, disturbance
Fear
Grieving, anticipatory

(Continued)

BOX 3–1   NURSING DIAGNOSES ORGANIZED ACCORDING TO DIAGNOSTIC DIVISIONS (Continued)

Grieving, dysfunctional
Hopelessness
Personal Identity disturbance
Post-Trauma Response
Powerlessness
Rape-Trauma Syndrome
Rape-Trauma Syndrome: compound reaction
Rape-Trauma Syndrome: silent reaction
Relocation Stress Syndrome
Self Esteem, chronic low
Self Esteem, disturbance
Self Esteem, situational low
Spiritual Distress (distress of the human spirit)
Spiritual Well Being, potential for enhancement

Diagnostic Division: Elimination

Ability to excrete waste products

DIAGNOSES

Bowel Incontinence
Constipation
Constipation, colonic
Constipation, perceived
Diarrhea
Incontinence, functional
Incontinence, reflex
Incontinence, stress
Incontinence, total
Incontinence, urge
Urinary Elimination, altered patterns
Urinary Retention [acute/chronic]

Diagnostic Division: Food/Fluid

Ability to maintain intake of and utilize nutrients and liquids to meet physiologic needs

DIAGNOSES

Breastfeeding, effective
Breastfeeding, ineffective
Breastfeeding, interrupted
Fluid Volume deficit [active loss]
Fluid Volume deficit [regulatory failure]
Fluid Volume deficit, risk for
Fluid Volume excess

(Continued)

BOX 3–1 NURSING DIAGNOSES ORGANIZED ACCORDING TO DIAGNOSTIC DIVISIONS (Continued)

Infant Feeding Pattern, ineffective
Nutrition, altered, less than body requirements
Nutrition, altered, more than body requirements
Nutrition, altered, risk for more than body requirements
Oral Mucous Membranes, altered
Swallowing, impaired

Diagnostic Division: Hygiene

Ability to perform activities of daily living

DIAGNOSES

Self Care deficit (specify): feeding, bathing/hygiene, dressing/grooming, toileting

Diagnostic Division: Neurosensory

Ability to perceive, integrate, and respond to internal and external cues

DIAGNOSES

Confusion, acute
Confusion, chronic
Infant Behavior, disorganized
Infant Behavior, disorganized, risk for
Infant Behavior, organized, potential for enhancement
Memory, impaired
Peripheral Neurovascular dysfunction, risk for
Sensory-Perceptual alterations (specify): visual, auditory, kinesthetic, gustatory, tactile, olfactory
Thought Processes, altered
Unilateral Neglect

Diagnostic Division: Pain/Discomfort

Ability to control internal/external environment to maintain comfort

DIAGNOSES

Pain [acute]
Pain, chronic

Diagnostic Division: Respiration

Ability to provide and use oxygen to meet physiologic needs

DIAGNOSES

Airway Clearance, ineffective
Aspiration, risk for
Breathing Pattern, ineffective
Gas Exchange, impaired

(Continued)

BOX 3–1 NURSING DIAGNOSES ORGANIZED ACCORDING TO DIAGNOSTIC DIVISIONS (Continued)

Spontaneous Ventilation, inability to sustain
Ventilatory Weaning Response, dysfunctional (DVWR)

Diagnostic Division: Safety

Ability to provide safe, growth-promoting environment

DIAGNOSES

Body Temperature, altered, risk for
Environmental Interpretation Syndrome, impaired
Health Maintenance, altered
Home Maintenance Management, impaired
Hyperthermia
Hypothermia
Infection, risk for
Injury, risk for
Perioperative Positioning Injury, risk for
Physical Mobility, impaired
Poisoning, risk for
Protection, altered
Self-Mutilation, risk for
Skin Integrity, impaired
Skin Integrity, impaired, risk for
Suffocation, risk for
Thermoregulation, ineffective
Tissue Integrity, impaired
Trauma, risk for
Violence, risk for, directed at self/others

Diagnostic Division: Sexuality

[Component of Ego Integrity and Social Interaction] Ability to meet requirements/characteristics of male/female role

DIAGNOSES

Sexual Dysfunction
Sexuality Patterns, altered

Diagnostic Division: Social Interaction

Ability to establish and maintain relationships

DIAGNOSES

Caregiver Role Strain
Caregiver Role Strain, risk for
Communication, impaired, verbal
Community Coping, enhanced, potential for
Community Coping, ineffective

(Continued)

BOX 3–1 NURSING DIAGNOSES ORGANIZED ACCORDING TO DIAGNOSTIC DIVISIONS (Continued)

Family Coping, ineffective: compromised
Family Coping, ineffective: disabling
Family Coping: potential for growth
Family Process, altered: Alcoholism
Family Processes, altered
Lonliness, risk for
Parent/Infant/Child Attachment, altered, risk for
Parental Role conflict
Parenting, altered
Parenting, altered, risk for
Role Performance, altered
Social Interaction, impaired
Social Isolation

Diagnostic Division: Teaching/Learning

Ability to incorporate and use information to achieve healthy lifestyle/optimal wellness

DIAGNOSES

Growth and Development, altered
Health-Seeking Behaviors (specify)
Knowledge deficit [Learning need] (specify)
Noncompliance [Compliance, altered] (specify)
Therapeutic Regimen: Community, ineffective management
Therapeutic Regimen: Families, ineffective management
Therapeutic Regimen: Individual, effective management
Therapeutic Regimen: Individual, ineffective management

BOX 3–2 WALKING THROUGH THE USE OF DIAGNOSTIC DIVISIONS

During the Assessment phase, the following data were obtained from Robert.

Activity/Rest

REPORTS (SUBJECTIVE)

Occupation: Retired truck driver
Usual Activities/Hobbies: Used to like to hunt
Leisure Time Activities: Mostly watch baseball on TV, take short walks— one to two blocks
Feelings of Boredom/Dissatisfaction: "Wish I could do more; just getting too old"
Limitations Imposed by Condition: "I get short of breath; stay at home mostly"

(*Continued*)

BOX 3–2 WALKING THROUGH THE USE OF DIAGNOSTIC DIVISIONS (Continued)

Sleep: Hours: 5   *Naps:* After lunch   *Aids:* None
  Insomnia: Only if short of breath (1 or 2×/wk) or needs to void (1×/night)
  Rested on Awakening: Not always; "feel weak most of the time"
  Other: "Sometimes it feels like there isn't enough air"

EXHIBITS (OBJECTIVE)

Observed Response to Activity: Cardiovascular: BP 178/102, P 100 after walking half length of corridor from floor scale
  Respiratory: 32, rapid, leaning forward to "catch breath"
Mental Status (i.e., withdrawn/lethargic): alert, responding to all questions
Neuromuscular Assessment: Muscle mass/tone: decreased, bilaterally equal/diminished   *Posture:* leans forward to breathe
Tremors: No   *ROM:* Movement in all extremities   *Strength:* moderate
  Deformity: No

Having previously noted respiratory cues of dyspnea with activity when you reviewed the Respiratory data in Box 2–5, you return to the Activity/Rest section of the Diagnostic Divisions, where the effects/limitations of this condition on both activity and sleep would also be considered. You are referred to the following nursing diagnoses Activity Intolerance [specify level]; Activity Intolerance, risk for, Disuse Syndrome, risk for; Diversional Activity deficit; Fatigue; and Sleep Pattern disturbance as possible choices to describe or label Robert's problem.

---

or be totally unrelated. In fact, cues may have relevance in more than one section, as you can see in Box 3–2.

STEP 2: RULE-OUT PROCESS

Alternative explanations are considered for the identified cues to determine which nursing diagnosis label may be the most appropriate. This step is crucial to establish an adequate list of diagnostic statements. As you compare and contrast the relationships among and between data, etiologic factors are identified within or between categories based on an understanding of the biologic, physical, and behavioral sciences.

> **For example:** Although *Hyperthermia* or *Infection, risk for*, were suggested during the first step of diagnostic reasoning, another consideration might be *Fluid Volume deficit*. In another example, cues of increased tension, restlessness, elevated pulse rate, and reported apprehension may initially be thought to indicate *Anxiety [specify level]*. However, a similar diagnosis of *Fear* should be considered, as well as the possibility that these cues may be physiologically based, needing medical treatment and nursing interventions related to learning needs/monitoring.

BOX 3-3   QUESTIONS TO ASK YOURSELF WHEN THE NURSING DIAGNOSIS LABEL IS UNCLEAR

When the nursing diagnosis label is unclear, you can ask yourself these questions:

1. What are my concerns about this patient?
2. Can I/am I doing something about it?
3. Can the overall risk be reduced by nursing intervention?
   For example, in the pediatric patient, fever is often a major concern. Questions to ask might be:

- What are the concerns about the fever?
  The patient may convulse.
- Can I do something about it?
  Try to bring the temperature down and make the environment safe.
- Can the overall risk be reduced by nursing interventions?
  Yes, the risk of convulsions can be reduced, if the temperature is lowered; or if convulsions do occur, measures can be taken to protect the patient from injury.

Conclusion: The Nursing Diagnosis would be Risk for Injury; and, the patient diagnostic statement would be Risk for Injury: seizure activity risk factor of prolonged high fever.

BOX 3-4   ELEMENTS OF NANDA NURSING DIAGNOSTIC LABELS

Appendix A supplies a complete listing of NANDA nursing diagnosis labels, which will be helpful to you as you work through the exercises in this chapter and throughout the book. It is important to become familiar with this list, so that you can find information quickly in the clinical setting. Take a moment to identify the key elements of the diagnostic label, "Fluid Volume deficit," as excerpted below.

Fluid Volume Deficit

Definition: The state in which an individual experiences vascular, cellular, or intracellular dehydration.
Related Factors: Active loss.
Defining Characteristics: Decreased urine output, output greater than intake, concentrated urine, sudden weight loss, decreased venous filling, hemoconcentration, increased serum sodium, thirst, hypotension, decreased skin turgor, increased pulse rate, dry skin/mucous membranes, increased body temperature, weakness, decreased pulse volume/pressure, change in mental state.
Now refer to Appendix A and locate the diagnosis Coping, Individual, ineffective. The graphic character "·" identifies the following as major or critical defining characteristics:

- Verbalization of inability to cope or inability to ask for help.
- Inability to problem solve.

When designated as major or critical characteristics in the nursing diagnosis, one or more of these cues must be present to confirm the correctness of the diagnosis for your patient.

If you encounter difficulty in choosing a nursing diagnosis label, the questions in Box 3–3 may provide additional guidance.

STEP 3: SYNTHESIZING THE DATA

Looking at all the data as a whole (including information collected by other members of the healthcare team) can provide a comprehensive picture of the patient in relation to the past, present, and future health status. This is called SYNTHESIZING the data. The suggested nursing diagnosis label is combined with the identified related factor(s) and cues to create a hypothesis.

> **For example:** Sally had a period of bleeding during delivery of the placenta following the unexpected delivery of twins. Blood loss was estimated to be approximately 600 mL. The nursing diagnosis label *Fluid Volume deficit [active loss]*; related factor, hemorrhage; cues, dark urine, dry mouth/lips, low blood pressure.

STEP 4: EVALUATING OR CONFIRMING THE HYPOTHESIS

Test the hypothesis for appropriate fit; that is, review the NANDA nursing diagnosis and definition. Then, compare the assessed possible ETIOLOGY with NANDA's RELATED FACTORS or RISK FACTORS. Next, compare the assessed patient cues with NANDA's Defining Characteristics, paying special attention to critical or major defining characteristics that should be present for the diagnosis to be confirmed. The addition of minor characteristics, if assessed, are used to support and provide an increased level of confidence in your selected nursing diagnosis. Appendix A provides a complete listing of NANDA nursing diagnostic labels, definitions, defining characteristics, and related factors. This listing will be helpful as you work through the Practice Activities and Work Pages contained in each chapter. Take a moment to review Box 3–4. The information contained within the box provides a beginning effort in assessing the appropriateness of a specific nursing diagnosis label.

Lunney (1989, 1990) addressed the self-monitoring task of accuracy determination and has defined characteristics of accuracy and an ordinal scale for measurement. The scale ranges from a high assigned accuracy point value describing a diagnosis that is consistent with all of the cues, to the lowest point value describing a diagnosis indicated by more than one cue but recommended for rejection based on the presence of at least two disconfirming cues (see Appendix E). Additionally, Appendix F, Lunney's Integrated Model for Self-Monitoring of Accuracy of the Diagnostic Process, is an excellent self-evaluation of your progress in diagnostic efforts. The completed evaluation provides feedback of your diagnostic abilities. Reflection and self-monitoring are tools to assist you in developing your *critical thinking* skills. The attention you give to measuring the accuracy of your suggested nursing diagnosis is time well spent. Comparing the subjective and objective data gathered from the patient with the defining characteristics of the possible nursing diagnosis that are listed not only helps to ensure the accuracy of your statement, but also stresses the importance of objectivity in this diagnostic process.

SYNTHESIZING—viewing all data as a whole to provide a comprehensive picture of the patient.

ETIOLOGY—identified causes and/or contributing factors responsible for the presence of a specific patient problem/need.

RELATED FACTOR—the conditions/circumstances that contribute to the development/maintenance of a nursing diagnosis; forms the "related to" component of the patient diagnostic statement.

RISK FACTOR—environmental factors and physiological, psychological, genetic, or chemical elements that increase the vulnerability of an individual, family, or community to an unhealthy event.

PRACTICE ACTIVITY 3–1

Record the cues relevant to the problem of Activity Intolerance, identified for Robert, in the appropriate spaces on this worksheet.

INTERACTIVE CARE PLAN WORKSHEET

Student Name:

ACTIVITY INTOLERANCE

Patient's Medical Diagnosis:

DEFINITION:	A state in which an individual has insufficient physiological or psychological energy to endure or complete required or desired daily activities.
DEFINING CHARACTERISTICS:	Verbal report of fatigue or weakness; abnormal heart rate or blood pressure response to activity; exertional discomfort or dyspnea; ECG changes reflecting dysrhythmias or ischemia.
RELATED FACTORS:	Bedrest and/or immobility; generalized weakness; sedentary life-style; imbalance between oxygen supply and/or demand.
STUDENT INSTRUCTIONS:	In the space below enter the subjective and objective data gathered during your patient assessment.

A S S E S S M E N T

Subjective Data Entry

Objective Data Entry

TIME OUT!

Student Instructions: To be sure your patient diagnostic statement written below is accurate, you need to review the defining characteristics and related factors associated with the nursing diagnosis, **Activity Intolerance**, and see how your patient data matches. Do you have an accurate match or is additional data required or does another nursing diagnosis need to be investigated?

D I A G N O S I S

PATIENT DIAGNOSTIC STATEMENT:

Activity Intolerance (specify) _____

_____

Related to _____

_____

Now return to Box 3–2. In reviewing Robert's data base, you *sense* he may have a problem with activity. After reviewing the NANDA nursing diagnosis labels and their definitions, relevant to the Activity/Rest Diagnostic Division, you choose the label Activity Intolerance, risk for. Next, to confirm your hypothesis, compare the cues from the data base with the related factors and defining characteristics noted in Appendix A. Practice Activity 3–1 presents an Interactive Care Plan Worksheet for the patient problem of Activity Intolerance, on which you can document the identified cues.

STEP 5: LIST THE PATIENT'S PROBLEMS/NEEDS

Based on the data obtained from steps 3 and 4, the accurate nursing diagnosis label is combined with the assessed etiology and signs/symptoms, if present, to finalize the patient diagnostic statement.

For example, Sally is diagnosed with a Fluid Volume deficit related to hemorrhage as evidenced by dark urine, dry mucous membranes, hypotension, and hemoconcentration. This individualized diagnosis reflects the P E S format for a three-part diagnostic statement, as described in Box 3–5. A diagnostic statement will be needed for *each* problem/need you identify. Take a moment here to complete Practice Activity 3–2.

STEP 6: REEVALUATE THE PROBLEM LIST

Be sure all areas of concern are noted. Once all nursing diagnoses are identified, list them according to priority and classify them according to status: An active problem/need; a risk or potential problem/need; or a resolved problem/need. Box 3–6 explains this status classification.

- *Active Diagnoses:* have already occurred and require some form of current action or intervention.

    For example: A patient is admitted for a medical workup for problems with bladder function related to her diagnosis of multiple sclerosis. An active problem might be Urinary Retention.

- *Risk or Potential Diagnoses:* may occur/recur, especially if intervention of some kind is not done to prevent them.

    For example: The patient's multiple sclerosis has been in remission, however, she has had difficulty in the past with physical mobility. This past problem must be considered when planning this patient's care in order to minimize the possibility of recurrence. A potential problem would then be identified as Physical Mobility, impaired, risk for.

- *Resolved Diagnoses:* are those that no longer need action.

    For example: Your patient once suffered a decubitus ulcer (Skin Integrity, impaired); however, she has learned techniques to prevent recurrence of this problem, and her skin is in good condition. Therefore, as long as she is able to participate in or direct her own care, this is of no significant concern to you at this time.

Finally, validate the diagnostic conclusions/impressions with the patient and/or a colleague. This helps to reduce the possibility of **DIAGNOSTIC ERRORS**

DIAGNOSTIC ERROR—a mistaken assumption leading to a wrong conclusion.

BOX 3–5 COMPONENTS OF THE PATIENT DIAGNOSTIC STATEMENT: PROBLEM, ETIOLOGY, AND SIGNS AND SYMPTOMS (P E S)

P = Problem/Need is the name or diagnostic label identified from the NANDA list. The key to accurate nursing diagnosis is problem identification that focuses attention on a current, risk or potential physical or behavioral response that interferes with the patient's quality of life. It deals with concerns of the patient/significant other(s) and the nurse, which require nursing intervention and management.

E = Etiology is the suspected cause or reason for the response that has been identified from the assessment (patient data base). The nurse makes inferences based on knowledge and expertise, such as understanding of pathophysiology, and situational or developmental factors. The etiology is stated as "related to." Note: One problem may have several suspected causes, such as Self Esteem disturbance, related to lack of positive feedback and dysfunctional family system.

S = Signs and Symptoms are the manifestations (or cues) identified in the assessment that substantiate the nursing diagnosis. They are stated as "evidenced by" followed by a list of subjective and objective data. It is important to note that *risk* or potential diagnoses are not accompanied by signs and symptoms because the problem has not yet actually occurred. In this instance, the "S" component of the problem statement is omitted and the "E" component would be replaced by an itemization of the identified risk factors which suggest that the diagnosis could occur. For example: Infection, risk for, risk factors of malnutrition, and invasive procedures.

BOX 3–6 STATUS CLASSIFICATION OF PATIENT PROBLEMS/NEEDS

- **Active:** A problem/need that is currently present and manifested by signs and symptoms. In recording the problem/need, you use a three-part P E S statement. Urinary Elimination, altered, related to sensory motor impairment evidenced by dribbling, 250 mL residual urine.
- **Risk or Potential:** A problem/need that you believe could develop, but because it has not yet occurred, there are no signs or symptoms, only "risk factors." The problem/need would be written as a two-part statement. Physical Mobility, impaired risk for, risk factors of neuromuscular impairment, decreased strength, and pain with movement.
- **Resolved:** A problem/need which no longer requires intervention. Because the problem no longer exists, no diagnostic statement is needed.

PRACTICE ACTIVITY 3–2

IDENTIFYING THE P E S COMPONENTS OF THE PATIENT DIAGNOSTIC STATEMENT

Instructions (questions 1–5): Identify the "P E S" components of each of these diagnostic statements:

1. Anxiety, severe, related to changes in health status of fetus/self and threat of death as evidenced by restlessness, tremors, focus on self/fetus.

   P = _____   E = _____   S = _____

2. Thought Processes, altered, related to pharmacologic stimulation of the nervous system as evidenced by altered attention span, disorientation, and hallucinations.

   P = _____   E = _____   S = _____

3. Coping, Individual, ineffective, related to maturational crisis as evidenced by inability to meet role expectations and alcohol abuse.

   P = _____   E = _____   S = _____

4. Hyperthermia related to increased metabolic rate and dehydration as evidenced by elevated temperature, flushed skin, tachycardia, and tachypnea.

   P = _____   E = _____   S = _____

5. Pain, acute, related to tissue distention and edema as evidenced by verbal reports, guarding behavior, and changes in vital signs.

   P = _____   E = _____   S = _____

6. Explain the difference between active and risk diagnoses: _____
   _____

7. Give an example of an active and a risk problem for a patient with second-degree burns of the hand. _____
   _____
   _____

and/or omissions as discussed in Box 3–7. Inclusion of the patient/significant others promotes understanding and participation in the planning of individualized care.

As you can see, the process of problem identification is more complex than simply attaching a label to your patient. In reviewing the definition of nursing, "the human responses to health problems" are complex and the process of accurately diagnosing these human responses attests to the complexity of nursing.

BOX 3-7 POTENTIAL ERRORS IN CHOOSING A NURSING DIAGNOSIS

- **Overlooking Cues** resulting in a missed diagnosis can lead to worsening of the problem.

  For example: A patient reports discomfort at the insertion site of an intravenous catheter (IV). You notice the area is slightly reddened but fail to consider the risk for infection. As a result, the patient develops sepsis or a blood infection requiring emergency intervention.

- **Making a Diagnosis with an Insufficient Data Base** can lead in the wrong direction, wasting valuable time and resources.

  For example: The patient displays signs of anxiety. Without additional assessment, you administer a tranquilizer on the belief that the signs and symptoms are psychologically based. Later, when checking the patient, you find signs of cyanosis, suggesting inadequate oxygenation. Thus, the anxiety probably was at least in part physiologically based and needed other nursing interventions.

- **Stereotyping** leads to treating all patients in the same way and negates individualization.

  For example: In a medical-surgical setting, the assumption is often made that a patient with a psychiatric diagnosis is apt to become violent.

Other Considerations for Problem Identification

The medical/psychiatric diagnosis can provide a starting point for identifying associated patient problems (problem sensing). Review Box 3–8 (see page 60) for several medical/psychiatric diagnoses with examples of associated nursing diagnoses. While they can suggest several nursing diagnoses, these nursing diagnoses must be supported by cues in the patient data base.

> **For example:** In the presence of a myocardial infarction, the patient often suffers pain, anxiety, and activity intolerance and requires teaching activities. In addition, the patient may be at risk for alteration of cardiac output, tissue perfusion, and fluid volume excess. These problems and needs are not necessarily present in each patient with this condition. One patient may actually be pain-free, whereas another could demonstrate a sleep disturbance or report spiritual distress. Therefore, a medical diagnosis can be an initial point for problem-sensing, but the validity of a nursing diagnosis depends on the presence of individually appropriate supporting data.

The patient's or family member's understanding of normal body function, individual expectations, or mistaken perceptions may result in the belief that a problem exists, even in the absence of diagnostically appropriate supporting data. Even though the problem seems to exist only in the mind of the patient/significant other, it needs to be addressed and resolved in order to promote optimal wellness.

For example:

1. The parent of a child with cancer may believe that the child is incapable of self-care activities even though the child's level of function and development would indicate otherwise. This then is not a patient problem with self-care but rather the parent's problem—possibly, Family Coping, ineffective: compromised.

2. A female patient may believe that sexual desire normally disappears after menopause/hysterectomy, and the fact that it has not, indicates to her that something is wrong. Although sexual dysfunction may have occurred, the assessment reveals inadequate information and misconceptions. Therefore, the nursing diagnosis is Knowledge deficit: normal sexual functioning.

3. An elderly, confused patient, with a diagnosis of Alzheimer's disease, is found wandering in the day room. She has soiled herself and is smearing feces on the walls and couch. The problem would not be one of bowel elimination but of Thought Processes, altered. Interventions would be addressed to the solution of behavioral management rather than only to a bowel control program.

As noted in the previous examples, it is important to "reduce" the problem to its basic component in order to focus interventions on the "roots" of the human response. It is also important to take the related factors as well as the defining characteristics to the lowest "denominator" possible so the patient and nurse are better able to formulate individually specific goals/outcomes and to identify more clearly the appropriate interventions/actions to be taken to correct or alleviate the problem.

For example: Social Interaction, impaired: related to neurologic impairment and the resulting sequelae (i.e., cognitive, behavioral, and emotional changes) is better stated, "related to skill deficit about ways to enhance mutuality, communication barriers, limited physical mobility as evidenced by family report of change in pattern of interacting, dysfunctional interactions with peers and family, observed discomfort in social situations." This simplifies care and increases the likelihood of a timely and satisfactory resolution.

Neurologic impairment is a broad umbrella that reflects general pathophysiology and lacks the specificity that is necessary to guide nursing actions/interventions. By identifying specific responses, you focus attention directly on issues that can be corrected or altered by nursing interventions.

As beginners, it is advisable to use the NANDA list in Appendix A when choosing a diagnostic label. Because the list is still in a state of evolution, however, "holes" may exist. With practice and experience, you may very well identify a problem or need that is treatable with nursing interventions but for which there is no appropriate NANDA label. In this situation, the diagnosis should be stated clearly using the P E S format and then reviewed with other nursing colleagues to verify that the meaning and intent are accurately communicated. Finally, the work should be documented and submitted to NANDA for consideration.

BOX 3–8 APPLICABLE NURSING DIAGNOSES ASSOCIATED WITH SELECTED MEDICAL/PSYCHIATRIC DISORDERS

Certain nursing diagnoses may be linked to specific health problems (e.g., medical disorders). This linkage is often presented as choices in a diagnostic data base, in various types of clinical pocket manuals, or on preprinted or computerized care planning forms. The purpose is to assist in rapidly identifying other applicable nursing diagnoses, based on the changing needs of the patient; and to develop a decisive plan of care.

Because the nursing process is cyclical and ongoing, other nursing diagnoses may become appropriate, as the individual patient situation changes. Therefore, you must continually assess, identify, and validate new problems and evaluate the effectiveness of subsequent care.

AIDS (Acquired Immunodeficiency Syndrome)

Infection, risk for*, progression to sepsis/opportunistic overgrowth risk factors may include suppressed inflammatory response and immunosuppression in combination with inadequate primary defenses, malnutrition, and environmental exposure.

Fluid Volume deficit, risk for*, risk factors may include excessive losses: copious diarrhea, profuse sweating, vomiting, hypermetabolic state, and fever; restricted intake: nausea and anorexia; lethargy.

Fatigue may be related to decreased metabolic energy production, increased energy requirements (hypermetabolic state), overwhelming psychologic/emotional and increased body temperature possibly evidenced by inability to maintain usual routines, decreased performance, lethargy/listlessness, and disinterest in surroundings.

Labor Stage I

Pain [acute/Discomfort], may be related to contraction-related hypoxia, dilation of tissues, and pressure on adjacent structures combined with stimulation of both parasympathetic and sympathetic nerve endings, possibly evidenced by verbal reports, distraction/guarding behaviors, and narrowed focus.

Urinary Elimination, altered may be related to retention of fluid in the prenatal period, increased glomerular filtration rate, decreased adrenal stimulation, dehydration, pressure of the presenting part, and regional anesthesia, possibly evidenced by increased/decreased output, decreased circulating blood volume, spasms of glomeruli and albuminuria, and reduced sensation.

Coping, Individual/Couple, ineffective, risk for,* risk factors may include stressors accompanying labor, use of ineffective coping mechanisms, and pain.

Fractures

Pain [acute] may be related to movement of bone fragments, muscle spasms, tissue trauma/edema, traction/immobility device, stress, and anxiety, possibly evidenced by verbal reports, distraction be-

(Continued)

BOX 3-8 APPLICABLE NURSING DIAGNOSES ASSOCIATED WITH SELECTED MEDICAL/PSYCHIATRIC DISORDERS (Continued)

haviors, self-focusing/narrowed focus, facial mask of pain, guarding/protective behavior, alteration in muscle tone, and autonomic responses.

Knowledge deficit [Learning need] (specify) regarding healing process, therapy requirements, and potential complications, may be related to lack of information, possibly evidenced by statements of concern, questions, and misconceptions.

Physical Mobility, impaired may be related to neuromuscular skeletal impairment, pain/discomfort, and restrictive therapies, possibly evidenced by inability to purposefully move within the physical environment, imposed restrictions, reluctance to attempt movement, limited range of motion, and decreased muscle strength/control.

Depressive Disorders (Mood Disorders)

MAJOR DEPRESSION, DYSTHYMIA

Violence, high risk for*, directed at self/others, risk factors may include depressed mood and feelings of worthlessness and hopelessness.

Coping, Individual, ineffective may be related to personal vulnerability, inadequate support systems, unrealistic perceptions, multiple life changes, inadequate coping method, unmet expectations, and actual/perceived loss possibly evidenced by perception of events and stressors in a manner that precipitates depressive episode, perception of areas in life as unfulfilled or as losses, denial of loss, verbalization of inability to cope or ask for help, expression of guilt, crying/labile affect, and chronic anxiety/depression.

Sleep Pattern, disturbance may be related to biochemical alterations (decreased serotonin levels), unresolved fears and anxieties, and inactivity possibly evidenced by difficulty in falling/remaining asleep, early morning awakening, reports of not feeling well rested, dark circles under eyes.

*A high-risk diagnosis is not evidenced by signs and symptoms as the problem has not occurred and nursing interventions are directed at prevention.

Extracted from Doenges and Moorhouse: Nurse's Pocket Guide, F.A. Davis, Philadelphia, 1993.

Nursing knowledge is both objective and subjective, and it is the combination of intuition and analysis that is nursing's methodology. Experienced nurses may use INTUITION to arrive at a conclusion as an integral part of critical thinking. This skill is difficult to teach, and may not develop in all nurses; however, it needs to be respected, valued, and encouraged. Intuition is grounded in both knowledge and experience and is involved in making nursing judgments. Paying attention to the feelings or sense of something for which there is no visible data can add an important dimension to the diagnostic reasoning process. Intuition, responsibly applied by checking, rechecking,

INTUITION—a sense of something that is not clearly evidenced by known facts.

BOX 3-9 QUALIFIERS FOR DIAGNOSTIC LABELS

(Suggested/not limited to the following)

Acute—Severe but of short duration.

Altered—A change from baseline.

Chronic—Lasting a long time; recurring; habitual; constant.

Decreased—Lessened, lesser in size, amount, or degree.

Deficient—Inadequate in amount, quality, or degree; defective; not sufficient; incomplete

Depleted—Emptied wholly or partially; exhausted of.

Disturbed—Agitated; interrupted, interfered with.

Dysfunctional—Abnormal; incomplete functioning.

Excessive—Characterized by an amount or quantity that is greater than is necessary, desirable, or useful.

Increased—Greater in size, amount or degree.

Impaired—Made worse, weakened; damaged, reduced; deteriorated.

Ineffective—Not producing in the desired effect.

Intermittent—Stopping and starting again at intervals; periodic; cyclic.

Potential for Enhanced (for use with wellness diagnoses)—Enhanced is defined as made greater, to increase in quality or more desired.

Types of Diagnostic Concepts

Actual—currently existing human response to health conditions/life processes that is supported by a cluster of defining characteristics (signs/symptoms) and include related factors (etiologies) that contribute to the development or maintenance of the diagnosis.

Risk—denotes a human response which *may* develop in a vulnerable person or group and is supported by risk factors that contribute to increased vulnerability.

Wellness—describes human responses to levels of wellness in an individual or group that have a potential for enhancement to a higher state.

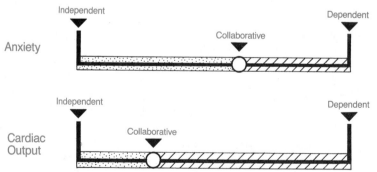

Figure 3-1. Representative comparison of the degree of independent nursing function in two nursing diagnoses. Nursing diagnoses have a varying degree of independent function, and nursing actions can be identified for any patient situation. As shown in this diagram, the nursing diagnosis *Anxiety* has a high degree of independent nursing actions, whereas *Cardiac Output* has a lower degree.

and validating these impressions (in order to avoid errors in judgment) can lead to insights not available in any other way.

Finally, problem identification may be assisted by entering the patient data base into a computer. On-line diagnostic software programs are available that contain lists of frequently used nursing diagnoses correlated to specific medical diagnoses. Other programs may suggest possible nursing diagnoses based on cues that the program identifies. Such programs are support tools and do not eliminate your need to use the diagnostic reasoning process to identify and formulate appropriate patient diagnostic statements *independently* of the computer recommendations.

WRITING A PATIENT DIAGNOSTIC STATEMENT: USING P E S

As NANDA's list of nursing diagnosis labels increases, and issues of **WELLNESS** are addressed, the focus of a nursing diagnosis may not be limited solely to problems but may also include the patient's needs and strengths as well. For this reason, although we use the P E S format, we have chosen to identify the outcome of the diagnostic reasoning process as the Patient Diagnostic Statement instead of the commonly used term *Patient Problem*.

WELLNESS—a state of optimal health, physical and psychosocial.

Using the P E S format as previously outlined, the problem/need, etiology, and signs and symptoms (or risk factors) are combined into a "neutral" statement avoiding value-laden or judgmental language. The use of ambiguous or judgmental terms such as, "too often," "uncooperative," or "manipulative," can lead to misunderstandings on the part of the reader. Patients may become defensive or other readers may be influenced to make an inaccurate or biased decision, resulting in a negative treatment outcome.

P E S—format for combining a patient problem label, etiology, and signs/symptoms to create an individualized diagnostic statement.

The *problem* and *etiology* sections of the diagnostic statement are joined by the phrase "related to." Phrases such as "due to" or "caused by" indicate a specific/limited causal link that should therefore be avoided. "Related to" suggests a connection between the nursing diagnosis and the identified factors, leaving open the possibility that there may be other contributing factors not yet recognized.

When writing a diagnostic statement, remember to include qualifiers or quantifiers as indicated in the NANDA list (e.g., Anxiety, severe . . .). If the term "specify" is noted with a diagnostic label, it is important that the correct information is provided to make the communication clear (review to Box 3–9).

> **For example:** Tissue perfusion, altered: *cerebral*; or Knowledge deficit regarding *care of the newborn*.

By definition, nursing diagnoses identify patient problems/needs that can be positively affected, or possibly prevented, by nursing actions. Some diagnoses permit greater independent function, whereas others are more collaborative. This may be visualized as a continuum without a fixed midpoint differentiating independent from dependent actions (Fig. 3–1). Furthermore, the extent of independent function is influenced by the individual nurse's experience, level of expertise, work setting, and presence of established **PROTOCOLS** or standards of care. For this reason, the authors recommend that nurses identify the nursing component and appropriate interventions for any patient

PROTOCOL—written guidelines of steps to be taken for providing patient care in a particular situation/ condition.

BOX 3–10 COMMON ERRORS IN CREATING AND WRITING THE PATIENT DIAGNOSTIC STATEMENT

Identifying an incorrect nursing diagnosis or misstatement of problems/needs can lead to incorrect goals/outcomes and inappropriate nursing interventions. This can result in inappropriate/inadequate treatment of the patient that may not resolve the problem and which may, on occasion, place the nurse at risk for legal liability.

- **Using the Medical Diagnosis:** Self Care deficit related to stroke.
  Correct: Self Care deficit related to neuromuscular impairment.
- **Relating the Problem to an Unchangeable Situation:** Injury, high risk for, related to blindness.
  Correct: Injury, risk for, related to unfamiliarity with surroundings.
- **Confusing the Etiology or Signs/Symptoms for the Problem:** Postoperative lung congestion related to bedrest.
  Correct: Airway Clearance, ineffective, related to general weakness and immobility.
- **Use of a Procedure Instead of the "Human Response":** Catheterization related to urinary retention.
  Correct: Urinary Retention related to perineal swelling.
- **Lack of Specificity:** Constipation related to nutritional intake.
  Correct: Constipation related to inadequate dietary bulk and fluid intake.
- **Combining Two Nursing Diagnoses:** Anxiety and Fear related to separation from parents.
  Correct: Fear related to separation from parents, or Anxiety, moderate, related to change in environment and unmet needs.
- **Relating One Nursing Diagnosis to Another:** Coping, Individual ineffective, related to anxiety.
  Correct: Anxiety, severe, related to change in role functioning and socioeconomic status.
- **Use of Judgmental/Value-Laden Language:** Pain, chronic, related to secondary/monetary gain.
  Correct: Pain, chronic, related to recurrent muscle spasms. **Note:** The patient's report is valid, but the issue of secondary gain may require additional assessment to choose other appropriate nursing diagnoses and interventions.
- **Making Assumptions:** Parenting altered, risk for, related to inexperience (new mother).
  Correct: Knowledge deficit regarding child care issues related to lack of previous experience, unfamiliarity with resources. **Note:** The label "Knowledge deficit" can have negative connotations for the patient and may result in defensive responses. The authors support the use of a substitute label "Learning Need."
- **Writing a Legally Inadvisable Statement:** Skin Integrity impaired, related to not being turned every 2 hours.
  Correct: Skin Integrity impaired, related to pressure and altered circulation. **Note:** If a patient complication occurs as a result of poor care/failure to meet standards of care, an incident report would be completed to document what happened.

problem, instead of labeling independent versus COLLABORATIVE PROBLEMS or potential complications.

For example:

- During and following Sally's bleeding episode, the nursing component would be *Fluid Volume deficit* [active loss] and the nurse would not only monitor the problem, but take action to control/prevent further blood loss (e.g., fundal massage) and would provide assurance to the patient.

- A low serum potassium level may result in dysrhythmias that can be addressed in *Cardiac Output, decreased, risk for*, requiring electro-cardiographic interpretation, possible limiting of activities, provision of potassium-containing foods/fluids as appropriate, and other interventions based on protocols.

- Michelle has a subclavian intravenous catheter. You might be concerned with *Infection, risk for*, with implications for sterile dressing changes and observation of the site.

There has been ongoing debate concerning the amount of independent function associated with nursing diagnoses and the interpretation of the definition of nursing diagnoses. These debates attest to the perceived and actual importance that nursing diagnoses have had and continue to have in the structuring of both the education and the practice of nursing.

Box 3–10 summarizes some common errors in creating and writing the patient diagnostic statement. Review this box and In a Nutshell before proceeding to Practice Activity 3–3 (see page 68).

COLLABORATIVE PROBLEM—*a need identified by another discipline that will contain a nursing component requiring nursing intervention and/or monitoring.*

SUMMARY

Although identifying an accurate nursing diagnosis requires time to analyze the gathered data and to validate the diagnosis, this process is critical and essential because it is the pivotal part of the nursing process. The time you take to formulate an accurate patient diagnostic statement and to plan the required care results in increased nursing efficiency, better use of time for all nursing staff, and the delivery of appropriate patient care, with the end result of better patient outcomes.

Some nurses still organize care directly around medical diagnoses, spending most of their time following medical orders. Medical diagnoses have a narrower focus than nursing diagnoses because they are based on pathology. A nursing diagnosis takes into account the psychological, social, spiritual, as well as physiological responses of the patient and family. NANDA diagnostic labels listed in Appendix A are used in formulating diagnostic statements that are structured in a three-part Problem, Etiology, and Signs/Symptoms (P E S) format. Two-part statements may be used for risk or potential diagnoses.

At times, what appears easy to do in theory may seem difficult to achieve in practice. Nurses often have visionary ideas for the delivery of quality care to all patients. All too frequently, turning those ideas into actions can seem to be a frustrating exercise in futility. However, as you work with and become more familiar with nursing diagnoses, the patient goals, related outcomes, and

IN A NUTSHELL . . .

How to Write a Patient Diagnostic Statement

1. Using physical assessment and history-taking interview techniques, collect both subjective and objective data from the patient, significant other, family members, other healthcare professionals, and patient records. A nursing framework is recommended such as Diagnostic Divisions (Doenges and Moorhouse), Functional Health Patterns (Gordon), or Human Response Patterns (NANDA).

2. Organize the collected data using a nursing framework (see item 1, above), a body systems approach (cardiovascular, gastrointestinal, and so on), a head-to-toe approach (head neck, thorax, and so on), or a combination of these. Your institution may use its own clustering model. If you have used a nursing framework, however, you will discover that information in the patient data base is already conveniently structured for ease in identifying applicable nursing diagnoses.

3. Using diagnostic reasoning skills, review and analyze the data base to identify cues (signs and symptoms) suggesting problems or needs that can be described by nursing diagnostic labels. Check the NANDA definitions of specific diagnoses for further assistance in distinguishing between two or more potentially applicable labels (see Appendix A).

4. Consider alternative rationales for the identified cues by comparing and contrasting the relationships among and between data, and isolating etiologic factors. This will allow you to determine which nursing diagnostic labels may be most appropriate, while ruling out those that are not.

5. Test your selection of nursing diagnostic label(s) and associated etiology(ies) for appropriate "fit" by:
   - Confirming the NANDA nursing diagnosis and definition for your choice of diagnostic label [P]
   - Comparing your proposed etiology with the NANDA "Related Factors" or "Risk Factors" associated with that particular diagnosis [E]
   - Comparing your identified signs and symptoms (cues) with the NANDA "Defining Characteristics" for the selected diagnosis, taking special note of the major/critical cues [S]

6. Re-evaluate your list of selected diagnoses to be sure that all patient problems/needs are accounted for. Then, order your list according to a needs priority model (the Maslow or Kalish models are usually used) and classify each diagnosis as active (signs and symptoms supporting it are already present), risk for (risk factors are present, but the problem has not yet occurred), or resolved (problem no longer requires nursing action).

7. Write the patient diagnostic statement for each diagnosis on your list. A three-part statement using the P E S format will be needed

(Continued)

> **IN A NUTSHELL . . . (Continued)**
>
> for active diagnoses, and an adaptation of the P E S format will be used to create the two-part statement needed for risk diagnoses. Resolved diagnoses do not require diagnostic statements.
>
> **Three-Part Patient Diagnostic Statement**
>
> To write the patient diagnostic statement for active diagnoses, combine (1) the confirmed nursing diagnosis label [P], (2) related factors [E], and (3) defining characteristics [S]. These elements are linked together by the phrases "related to" and "as evidenced by":
>
> PROBLEM: [nursing diagnostic label]
> ETIOLOGY: Related to [etiologic factors]
> SIGNS AND SYMPTOMS: As evidenced by [defining
>   characteristics]
>
> **Two-Part Diagnostic Statement**
>
> To write the diagnostic statement for risk diagnoses, combine (1) the confirmed risk nursing diagnosis label [P] and (2) the associated risk factors [E]. These elements are linked together by the phrase "risk factors of."
>
> PROBLEM: [risk nursing diagnosis label]
> ETIOLOGY: Risk factors of [associated risk factors]

nursing interventions for attaining these goals and outcomes become more readily apparent. As you can see, an accurate and complete nursing diagnosis serves as the basis for the activities of the *Planning* step of the nursing process, discussed in Chapter 4.

Before continuing, let us return to the second ANA Standard of Clinical Nursing Practice and review the measurement criteria necessary to achieve and ensure compliance with the standard as discussed in this chapter (Box 3–11).

PRACTICE ACTIVITY 3-3

IDENTIFYING CORRECT AND INCORRECT PATIENT DIAGNOSTIC STATEMENTS

Label each patient diagnostic statement as correct or incorrect. Identify why a statement is incorrect:

_____ 1. Airway Clearance, ineffective, related to increased pulmonary secretions and bronchospasm evidenced by wheezing, tachypnea, and ineffective cough. _____

_____ 2. Thought Processes, altered, related to delusional thinking or reality base evidenced by persecutory thoughts of "I am victim," and interference with ability to think clearly and logically. _____

_____ 3. Gas Exchange, impaired, related to bronchitis evidenced by rhonchi, dyspnea, and cyanosis. _____

_____ 4. Knowledge Deficit, diabetic care, related to inaccurate follow-through of instructions evidenced by information misinterpretation and lack of recall. _____

_____ 5. Pain, related to tissue distention and edema evidenced by reports of severe colicky pain in right flank, elevated pulse and respirations, and restlessness. _____

BOX 3-11   MEASUREMENT CRITERIA FOR ANA STANDARD II

ANA Standard II: Diagnosis: The nurse analyzes the assessment data in determining diagnoses.

1. Diagnoses are derived from the assessment data.
2. Diagnoses are validated with the patient, significant other(s), and healthcare providers.
3. Diagnoses are documented in a manner that facilitates the determination of expected outcomes and plan of care.

WORK PAGE: Chapter Three

1. What is the definition of Problem Identification? _____

_____

2. What two factors influenced the development and acceptance of nursing diagnosis as the language of nursing? _____

_____

_____

3. List three reasons for using nursing diagnosis:

a. _____

b. _____

c. _____

4. List the six steps of diagnostic reasoning:

a. _____

b. _____

c. _____

d. _____

e. _____

f. _____

5. Name the components of the Patient Diagnostic Statement:

a. _____

b. _____

c. _____

6. If a risk or potential problem is identified, how is the Patient Diagnostic Statement altered?

_____

_____

7. What is the difference between a medical and a nursing diagnosis? _____

_____

_____

8. Which of these patient diagnostic statements are stated correctly? Indicate by placing a C before correct, or an I before incorrect statements. Then, differentiate actual (A) from risk (R) problems by placing an A or R by each statement:

_____ a. Knowledge deficit, drug therapy related to misinterpretation and unfamiliarity with resources as evidenced by request for information and statement of misconception.

_____ b. Risk for Infection, risk factors of altered lung expansion, decreased ciliary action, decreased hemoglobin, and invasive procedures.

_____ c. Urinary Elimination, altered, related to indwelling catheter evidenced by inability to void.

_____ d. Anxiety [moderate], related to change in health status, role functioning, and socioeconomic status evidenced by apprehension, insomnia, and feelings of inadequacy.

9. Underline the cues in the patient data base below which indicate that a problem may exist, and write a Patient Diagnostic Statement based on your findings.

Vignette: Sally is 2 days' postdelivery. She reports her bowels have not moved but says she has been drinking plenty of fluids, including fruit juices and has been eating a balanced diet.

ELIMINATION (EXCERPT FROM THE PATIENT DATA BASE)

Subjective

Usual bowel patterns: every morning
Laxative use: rare/MOM PM
Character of stool: brown, formed
Last BM: 4 days ago
History of bleeding: No
Hemorrhoids: last 5 weeks
Constipation: since delivery
Diarrhea: No
Usual voiding pattern: 3–4 x/day
Incontinence: No
Urgency: No
Character of urine: Yellow
Pain/burning/difficulty voiding: No
History of kidney/bladder disease: several bladder infections, last one 6 years ago
Associated complaints: pain with stool, nausea, "I just can't go no matter what I do."

Objective

Abdomen tender: Yes
Soft/firm: somewhat firm
Palpable mass: No
Size/girth: enlarged/postpartal
Bowel sounds: present all four quadrants, hypoactive every 1 to 2 minutes

ELIMINATION (EXCERPT FROM THE PATIENT DATA BASE) (Continued)

Objective

Hemorrhoids: Visual examination not done

Now, write the Patient Diagnostic Statement. Refer to the listing of Nursing Diagnoses in Appendix A to compare diagnostic labels addressing bowel elimination.

_____

_____

_____

_____

_____

BIBLIOGRAPHY

American Nurses' Association. (1980). *Nursing: A Social Policy Statement.* Kansas City, MO: Author.

Briody, M.E., Carpenito, L.J., Jones, D.A., & Fitzpatrick, J.J. (1992). Toward further understanding of nursing diagnosis: An interpretation. *Nursing Diagnosis, 3*(3): 124–128.

Carpenito, L.J. (1992). *Nursing Diagnosis: Application to Clinical Practice* (5th ed.). Philadelphia: J.B. Lippincott.

Cassmeyer, V.L. (1989). Using physiology and pathophysiology in the nursing diagnosis process. *Journal of Advanced Medical-Surgical Nursing, 1*(3):1–10.

Fry, V.S. (1953). The creative approach to nursing. *American Journal of Nursing, 53*:301–302.

Gebbie, K.M., & Lavin, M.A. (1975). *Classification of Nursing Diagnoses: Proceeding From the First National Conference.* St. Louis, MO: Mosby.

Gordon, M. (1976). Nursing diagnosis and the diagnostic process. *American Journal of Nursing, 76*(8):1298–1300.

Gordon, M. (1993). *Nursing Diagnosis: Process and Application* (3rd ed.). St. Louis, MO: C.V. Mosby.

Kim, M.J. (1984). Physiologic nursing diagnosis: Its role and place in nursing taxonomy. In M.J. Kim, G.K. McFarland, & A.M. McLane (Eds.), *Classification of Nursing Diagnoses: Proceedings of the Fifth National Conference.* St. Louis, MO: C.V. Mosby.

Lunney, M. (1989). Self-monitoring of accuracy using an integrated model of diagnostic process. *Journal of Advanced Medical-Surgical Nursing, 1*(3)43–52.

Lunney, M. (1990). Accuracy of nursing diagnosis: Concept development. *Nursing Diagnosis, 1*(1):12–17.

Lunney, M. (1992). Divergent productive thinking factors and accuracy of nursing diagnoses. *Research in Nursing & Health, 15*(3):303–311.

Wallace, D., & Ivey, J. (1989). *The Bifocal Clinical Nursing Model: Descriptions and Applications to Patient's Receiving Thrombolytic or Anticoagulant Therapy, 4*(1): 33–45.

SUGGESTED READING

Advant, K.C. (1990). The art and science in nursing diagnosis development. *Nursing Diagnosis, 1*(1):51–56.

American Nurses' Association (1973). *Standards of Nursing Practice.* Kansas City, MO: Author.

American Nurses' Association (1991). *Standards of Clinical Nursing Practice.* Kansas City, MO: Author.

Carlson, J.H., Craft, C.A., & McGuire, A.D. (1982). *Nursing Diagnosis.* Philadelphia: W.B. Saunders.

Carnevali, D.L. (1983). *Nursing Care Planning: Diagnosis and Management.* Philadelphia: J.B. Lippincott.

Carnevali, D.L., Mitchell, P.H., Woods, N.F., & Tanner, C.A. (1984). *Diagnostic Reasoning in Nursing.* Philadelphia: J.B. Lippincott.

Carnevali, D.L., & Thomas, M.D. (1993). *Diagnostic Reasoning and Treatment Decision Making in Nursing.* Philadelphia: J.B. Lippincott.

Cox, H. et al. (1993). *Clinical Applications of Nursing Diagnosis: Adult Health, Child Health, Women's Health, Mental Health, and Home Health* (2nd ed.). Philadelphia: F.A. Davis.

Craft, M.J., & Denehy, J.A. (1990). *Nursing Interventions for Infants and Children.* Philadelphia: W.B. Saunders.

Doenges, M.E., Moorhouse, M.F., & Geissler, A.C. (1993). *Nursing Care Plans: Guidelines for Planning and Documenting Patient Care* (3rd ed.). Philadelphia: F.A. Davis.

Kerr, M. (1991). Validation of taxonomy. In R. Carrol-Johnson (Ed.), *Classification of Nursing Diagnoses: Proceedings of Ninth Conference* (pp. 6–13). Philadelphia: J.B. Lippincott.

Kerr, M. et al. (1992). Development of definitions for taxonomy II. *Nursing Diagnosis, 3*(2):65–71.

Kerr, M. et al. (1993). Taxonomic validation: An overview. *Nursing Diagnosis, 4*(1):6–14.

LeMone, P. (1993). Validation of the defining characteristics of altered sexuality. *Nursing Diagnosis, 4*(2):56–62.

Levin, R.F., Krainovich, B.C., Bahrenburg, E., & Mitchell, C.A. (1988). Diagnostic content validity of nursing diagnosis. *Image, 21*(1):40–44.

Leuner, J.D., Manton, A.K., Kelliher, D.B., Sullivan, S.B., & Doherty, M. (1990). *Mastering the Nursing Process: A Case Study Approach.* Philadelphia: F.A. Davis.

Loomis, M.E., & Conco, D. (1991). Patient's perception of health, chronic illness, and nursing diagnosis. *Nursing Diagnosis, 2*(4):162–170.

Maas, M., Buckwalter, K.C., & Hardy, M. (1991). *Nursing Diagnosis and Interventions for the Elderly.* Menlo Park, CA: Addison-Wesley.

Mahon, S.M. (1994). Concept analysis of pain: Implications related to nursing diagnoses. *Nursing Diagnosis, 1*(5):15–25.

Miers, L.J. (1991). NANDA's definition of nursing diagnosis: A plea for conceptual clarity. *Nursing Diagnosis, 2*(1):9–18.

Mills, W.C. (1991). Nursing diagnosis: The importance of a definition. *Nursing Diagnosis, 2*(1):3–8.

Minton, J.A., & Creason, N.S. (1991). Evaluation of admission nursing diagnoses. *Nursing Diagnosis, 2*(3):119–125.

North American Nursing Diagnosis Association. (1992). *NANDA Nursing Diagnoses: Definitions and Classification—1992.* St. Louis, MO: Author.

Shoemaker, J.K. (1984). Essential features of a nursing diagnosis. In M.J. Kim, G.K. McFarland, & A.M. McLane (Eds.) *Classification of Nursing Diagnoses: Proceedings of the Fifth National Conference.* St. Louis, MO: Mosby.

Warren, J.J., & Hoskins, L.M. (1990). The development of NANDA's nursing diagnosis taxonomy. *Nursing Diagnosis, 1*(4):162–168.

Whitley, G.G. (1992). Concept analysis of anxiety. *Nursing Diagnosis, 3*(3):107–116.

Whitley, G.G. (1992). Concept analysis of fear. *Nursing Diagnosis, 3*(4):155–161.

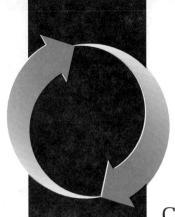

CHAPTER 4

The Planning Step: Creating the Plan of Care

ANA Standard 3: Outcome Identification: The nurse identifies expected outcomes individualized to the client.

ANA Standard 4: Planning: The nurse develops a plan of care that prescribes interventions to attain expected outcomes.

Once the etiology, signs, and symptoms previously identified are incorporated into a patient diagnostic statement, you can proceed to the PLANNING step of the nursing process. Now, attention is focused on the actions that are most appropriate to effectively address the patient's problems/needs. You begin to set priorities, establish goals, identify desired outcomes, and determine specific

PLANNING—third step of the nursing process during which goals/outcomes are determined and interventions chosen.

73

PLAN OF CARE—written evidence of the second and third steps of the nursing process that identifies the patient's problems/needs, goals/outcomes of care, and interventions to achieve the outcomes and treat the problems/need.

nursing interventions. These actions are documented as the **PLAN OF CARE**, which then serves to guide the activities of all healthcare workers who are involved in the patient's care. Whenever possible, the patient and/or significant others are included in the process of **PLANNING**, so that they may contribute to, participate in, and take responsibility for their own care and the achievement of the desired outcomes and goals.

SETTING PRIORITIES FOR PATIENT CARE

The starting point for planning care is to generally rank the patient's problems/needs, so that the nurse's attention and subsequent actions are properly focused. While there are many ways of prioritizing patient needs, a useful framework is one developed by Abraham Maslow (Fig. 4–1). In 1943, Maslow theorized that human behavior is motivated by a hierarchy arranged from basic to progressively higher-level needs. According to Maslow, physiologic needs are generally considered baseline survival needs because they must be met in order for life to continue. When these base-level needs (such as food, fluid, and oxygen) are not satisfied, it is difficult or impossible to focus on, or attempt to meet, higher-level needs (such as love, belonging, and self-esteem). Once base-level needs are satisfied, however, it becomes possible for higher-level needs to be addressed.

Richard Kalish expanded and further subdivided the structure of Maslow's hierarchy, resulting in a more comprehensive description of the specific need categories. This expanded hierarchy can help you, as a nurse, to identify and prioritize patient needs more precisely as well as desired outcomes and the associated nursing interventions (Fig. 4–2). Failure to meet human needs at any level can dramatically interfere with a patient's overall progress. Clearly, it is difficult to use Active Listening techniques (meeting a higher-level patient need for self-esteem) to teach a patient who is choking (a basic need of survival) about maintaining a patent airway.

Figure 4–1. Maslow's hierarchy of needs. The pyramid of Maslow's hierarchy is a model that allows us to look at human behavior in a structured way to determine physiological and psychological needs. Physiological needs appear at the bottom or base of the pyramid. Maslow's theory tells us that these lower-level needs must be met before higher-level needs (such as self-esteem) can be addressed. This knowledge of the needs that must be met first can help the nurse determine the priorities of patient care.

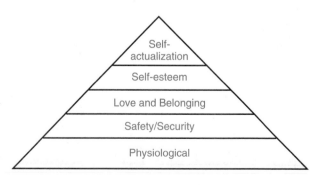

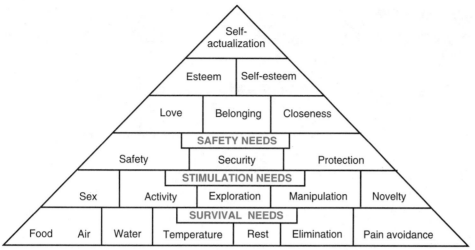

Figure 4–2. Kalish's expanded hierarchy. In an expansion of Maslow's model, Kalish restructured the first two levels of Maslow's pyramid (physiological and safety/security needs) into three levels and identified more-specific subcategories. The base level is labeled *survival*, the second level *stimulation*, and the third level *safety*. The refinement of these subcategories can further assist the nurse to identify the priorities for planning patient care.

Once you determine the priorities of care, the patient's care needs can be ranked, based on a system (such as Maslow's hierarchy; see Appendix C) that can help you identify basic to higher-level needs/actions. This is necessary because it is usually difficult to plan and provide care effectively when more than three to five patient problems exist at one time, depending on each problem's complexity. By ranking the patient's problems/needs, you can proceed in a logical way to facilitate your patient's recovery.

For example:

- Basic survival needs (i.e., air, water, and food) must be met before other needs can be considered. Sample diagnostic labels involving basic survival needs include Airway Clearance, ineffective, and Nutrition, altered, less than body requirements.

- Safety needs are next in order of importance. Nursing diagnostic labels relating to safety needs include Violence, risk for, directed at self/others; Injury, risk for; Health Maintenance, altered.

- Once these categories of patient care needs are met, concerns regarding needs in the social, self-esteem, and self-actualization categories can be considered. Examples of nursing diagnostic labels relating to these categories of needs are: Social Interaction, impaired (a need for relationships with others); Self Esteem disturbance (the need to feel good about oneself); and Family Coping: potential for growth (a need for family and belonging).

Setting priorities for patient care is a complex and dynamic challenge. What you may perceive as the number one patient care need or appropriate nursing intervention today could change tomorrow or for that matter within

PRACTICE ACTIVITY 4–1

PRIORITIZING NURSING DIAGNOSES

Instructions: Prioritize the nursing diagnoses listed in each separate set by using the Maslow and Kalish models. Rank the four diagnoses by using 1 to designate the most basic or more immediate patient need and continuing to 4, which designates the highest-level need (but least in priority). Review Appendix A as needed to compare definitions of these nursing diagnoses.

a. _____ Incontinence, stress
  _____ Sexuality Patterns, altered
  _____ Airway Clearance, ineffective
  _____ Skin Integrity, impaired, risk for

b. _____ Gas Exchange, impaired
  _____ Knowledge deficit
  _____ Hypothermia
  _____ Infection, risk for

c. _____ Pain, acute
  _____ Self Esteem, chronic low
  _____ Physical Mobility, impaired
  _____ Social Isolation

GOALS—broad guidelines indicating the overall direction for movement as a result of the interventions of the healthcare team; divided into long-term goals and short-term goals.

LONG-TERM GOALS—those goals that may not be achieved before discharge from care but may require continued attention by patient and/or others.

SHORT-TERM GOALS—those goals that usually must be met before discharge or movement to a less acute level of care.

minutes. Practice Activity 4–1 will give you some experience prioritizing patient problems based on levels of need.

Establishing Patient Goals

Once you have prioritized patient problems, establish the **GOALS** for treatment/discharge. The patient care goal(s) is a broad description of the general direction in which your patient is expected to progress in response to treatment.

Goals may be either long-term or short-term. **LONG-TERM GOALS** indicate the overall direction or end result of care and may very well *not* be achieved before discharge. Examples of long-term goals might be "Maintains control of blood glucose level" or "Uses resources/supports to prevent rehospitalization." **SHORT-TERM GOALS** are more specific guides for care and must usually be met before discharge or transfer to a less acute level of care, supervision, or support. Short-term goals may be building blocks for attaining the long-term goals. Nursing care can then be planned more accurately when the focus is directed to the short-term goals. Depending on the patient's anticipated length of stay/care, a short-term goal may be evaluated within a few hours or over the period of several therapeutic sessions. This period of time could reflect as much as several calendar weeks if the patient is seen for counseling/therapy on a weekly, or even monthly, basis. Examples of short-term goals might be "Learns to use blood glucose monitoring system" or "Using three support agencies within the community appropriately."

If the short-term goal is to be met within the nursing shift during which it is identified, it is not necessary to write the goal on the plan of care; it can be noted in the progress note. If the goal is not accomplished by the end of the shift, it is added to the plan of care, with a new timeframe, so that oncoming nurses can continue to work toward it.

Identifying Desired Outcomes

The next step in developing the plan of care is to form specific, OUTCOMES, which are defined as patient responses that are achievable and desired by the patient and that can be attained within a defined time period given the present situation and resources. These *desired outcomes* are the measurable steps toward achieving the patient goals that were established earlier. Because they must be measurable, outcome statements need to:

- Be specific
- Be realistic
- Consider the patient's circumstances and desires
- Indicate a definite timeframe
- Provide measurable evaluation criteria for determining success or failure

Desired outcomes are written by listing items/behaviors that can be observed and monitored to determine whether or not a positive/acceptable outcome has been achieved within the indicated timeframe. For example, "Verbalizes understanding of disease process and potential complications. . . ." This itemized listing of outcomes then serves as the evaluation tool, which will be discussed more fully in Chapter 6. Take a moment to look over Box 4–1 to give you a better idea of how to make the distinction between goals and outcomes.

Measurable action verbs are used to describe outcomes. Some examples of this type of verb are: discusses, states, identifies, administers, explains, and reports. For instance, "Patient will: *Ambulate* with use of cane." Refer to Box 4–2 for additional examples. Passive words are generally avoided. The use of specific time elements in outcome statements also provide measurable criteria, such as: "Patient will: Ambulate with cane without assistance *within 3 days*." On occasion, some outcomes may be ongoing because they do not have a specific timeframe, short of discharge from care. Examples of these ongoing outcomes would be statements such as "Patient will: Maintain a patent airway" or "Patient will: Be free of skin breakdown." It is your job to monitor each of these situations and document regularly any patient findings. However, the situations may not be *resolved* until the patient's condition/status changes or discharge has occurred.

When outcomes are properly written, they provide direction for planning and validating the choice of appropriate nursing interventions.

For example:

- Patient will: Identify individual nutritional needs within 30 hours.
- Patient will: Formulate a dietary plan based on these needs within 48 hours.

From these desired outcomes, you know that the patient's level of dietary knowledge should be assessed, individual patient needs identified, and pa-

OUTCOMES—measurable steps to achieve the goals of treatment and to meet discharge criteria; the result of actions undertaken to achieve a broader goal.

BOX 4–1   DISTINGUISHING BETWEEN GOALS AND OUTCOMES

Goals are overall, broad directions to guide the plan of care. A broad goal for a patient with chronic obstructive pulmonary disease (COPD) might be:

• Ventilation/oxygenation adequate to allow a functional lifestyle.

Outcomes are the desired results of actions undertaken to achieve the broader goal and are the measurable steps to achieving the goals of treatment/discharge criteria. Often there is more than one outcome for each goal. The integral outcomes to achieve the above goal could include:

• Maintains patent airway with breath sounds clear.
• Demonstrates techniques to improve airway clearance (i.e., use of pursed-lip breathing, liquifying secretions, and/or nebulizer therapy).
• Initiates necessary lifestyle changes and participates in treatment regimen.

---

tient teaching information presented to provide the patient with the tools necessary to formulate a dietary plan.

Remember, though, interventions can be wide ranging. The outcome statement "Patient will: Verbalize acceptance of actual body image within 2 weeks" may call for interventions ranging from learning to recognize and express own feelings about body changes; to developing a program of diet and exercise to promote weight loss; to instruction in the use of makeup, hairstyles, and ways of dressing that maximize figure assets.

BOX 4–2   ACTION VERBS USEFUL IN WRITING MEASURABLE OUTCOMES

Using action rather than passive verbs provides a clearer method to determine patient progress. The following are examples of action verbs that can be measured or observed.

> List, Record, Name, State
> Describe, Explain, Identify
> Demonstrate, Use, Schedule
> Differentiate, Compare, Relate
> Design, Prepare, Formulate
> Select, Choose, Compare
> Increase/Decrease, Stand, Walk, Participate

For example: The patient will: *List* three things he understands about his diagnosis. The patient will: *Walk* to the end of the hall and back three times today.

Below are a few samples of "passive" verbs. Notice that the "actions" described by the verbs are not measurable:

> Understand, Feel, Learn, Know, Accept

For example: The patient will: *Understand* his treatment plan. How will the nurse measure achievement and *know* that the patient understands?

All outcomes should tell the readers specifically what the patient is working on or doing. If the outcome does not seem to logically relate to the goals for treatment/discharge, it should be questioned. Is the outcome, in fact, a valid component of the plan of care? With this in mind, there is a simple and straightforward method of determining whether or not an outcome is correctly written: Ask yourself if you could observe the patient in the performance of the behavior indicated. If the answer is no, the desired, measurable outcome you have written should be modified. Below are several pairs of correctly and incorrectly written outcomes with notations to identify the desired elements. When you have finished looking them over, work through the exercises in Practice Activity 4–2.

1. **Incorrect:** "Understands insulin therapy within 48 hours."
   Rationale: This patient outcome states a clear time line, but can you measure a patient's "understanding"? This outcome needs a measurable action verb.
   Correct: "Demonstrates correct insulin administration techniques within 48 hours."
   or
   "Explains reasons for the steps of insulin administration within 48 hours."
   Rationale: These are well-written outcomes that are observable, measurable, and time limited.

2. **Incorrect:** "Requires no reminders from staff regarding dietary restrictions within 3 days."
   Rationale: This outcome tells what the staff will do, not what the patient will do.
   Correct: "Lists individual dietary restrictions and makes appropriate choices from daily menu within 3 days."
   Rationale: This outcome is observable and easy to document.

3. **Incorrect:** "Receives fewer restrictions for defying staff instructions during the next 2 weeks."
   Rationale: What exactly is the definition of "fewer"? A specific number is clearer. What constitutes "defiance," and what is the patient doing? According to this outcome, the patient "receives" fewer restrictions, which places the patient in an essentially passive role. Good measurable outcomes state what the patient actively does.
   Correct: "Follows rules so that infractions decrease from the current rate of five per week to no more than two per week within 7 days."
   Rationale: Incidents of violation of unit rules are events that are observable, well documented, and easy to track. This outcome is also time limited.

SELECTING APPROPRIATE NURSING INTERVENTIONS

NURSING INTERVENTIONS are prescriptions for behaviors, treatments, activities, or actions that assist the patient in achieving the expected outcomes. Nursing interventions, like nursing diagnoses, are key elements of the knowledge of nursing; in fact, the scientific body of knowledge of nursing interventions like that of nursing diagnoses continues to grow as research supports the connec-

NURSING INTERVENTIONS—any direct care treatment that a nurse performs on behalf of a patient, including nurse and physician-initiated treatments (resulting from nursing and medical diagnoses), and provision of essential daily functions for the patient who cannot do them (Bulechek & McCloskey, 1989).

PRACTICE ACTIVITY 4-2

IDENTIFYING CORRECTLY STATED OUTCOMES

Instructions: *Identify which of the following outcome statements are written correctly, or if not written correctly state why it is incorrect. Modify those statements that are not correct.*

1. Patient will: List individual risk factors and appropriate interventions. _____

_____

2. Patient will: Identify four adaptive/protective measures for individual situation by discharge.

_____

_____

3. Patient will: Understand behaviors, lifestyle changes necessary to promote physical safety

within 72 hours. _____

_____

4. Airway patent, aspiration prevented, ongoing. _____

_____

5. Patient will: Assume responsibility for own learning by participating in group discussions

twice a day no later than 10/29/95. _____

_____

tion between actions and outcomes. (McCloskey & Bulechek, 1992). In Chapter 3 we discussed the need to select the right nursing diagnosis. Selecting the appropriate nursing intervention so that your patient can achieve the desired outcomes is as important as accuracy in diagnosing. It also is another method of individualizing your patient's care.

Naturally your expectation is that the interventions you select will benefit the patient and/or significant other in a predictable way. You need to base your nursing interventions on the patient's nursing diagnosis, the established goals and desired outcomes, the ability of the nurse to successfully implement the intervention and the ability, appropriateness, and willingness of the patient to undergo the intervention. Interventions need to be age/situation appropriate and promote identified patient strengths, when possible.

For example:

- Discussion of fears may help to reduce the adult patient's level of anxiety, whereas an infant will respond more positively to *holding and cuddling.*

- Orange juice is a good choice for fluid replacement unless the patient has open lesions on the oral mucosa, in which case, mild fruit nectars would be preferred, as acidic juices will cause pain.

- Visualization to assist with stress or pain management may be the appropriate intervention for the patient assessed as having creative abilities.

You are accountable for being current and accurate when identifying nursing interventions. Therefore, you need to be familiar with the body of scientific knowledge (rationale) that supports these interventions.

NURSING STANDARDS and agency policy must also be considered when choosing specific interventions. For example, one nursing standard describes the minimum level for nursing care related to urinary catheterization. The standard also contains the policies and procedures required to meet the standard. The policy identifies the level of educational preparation that is required to perform the procedure while the procedural section provides the needed equipment and suggested method of performing the procedure. The interventions must be deliberate and purposeful and include independent nursing activities (such as frequency of monitoring activities/focused assessments, counseling, teaching, suctioning an airway), as well as any collaborative activities necessary to carry out orders from other healthcare providers (including consultation by and referral to other providers).

To be communicated accurately, nursing interventions, like nursing diagnoses and patient care goals and outcomes, need to be developed in the correct format and be specifically and clearly stated. The following criteria should be included in creating and documenting the intervention in the patient's plan of care:

- The date the intervention is written
- An action verb describing the activity to be performed
- Qualifiers of how, when, where, time/frequency, and amount
- Signature and/or initials of originating nurse

　　For example:

- 1/27 Assist as needed with self-care activities each AM. *AG*
- 6/12 Record respiratory and pulse rates before, during, and after activity. *BB*
- 3/13 Inspect wound during each dressing change. *MR*
- 10/12 Measure intake and output hourly. *SP*

Note: Depending on agency policy, when the original plan of care is written, a single date and signature is sufficient. As subsequent interventions are added, the entry should be individually dated and initialed or signed. Now take a moment to complete Practice Activity 4–3 before proceeding to Box 4–3, which walks you through the first three steps of the nursing process. Patient data are presented, and a patient problem is identified. Then a goal, outcomes, and appropriate interventions are chosen to treat the problem.

THE PATIENT PLAN OF CARE

Planning care can save valuable time when the goals of care, patient outcomes, and nursing interventions to achieve them are clearly identified, and then recorded, for all to see. The documentation of the planning process is the

PRACTICE ACTIVITY 4-3

IDENTIFYING CORRECTLY STATED INTERVENTIONS

Instructions: *Identify which of the following interventions are correctly stated, and rewrite those that are not.*

1. Walk length of hall 2 x/day with assistance from two staff members. _____

_____

2. Force fluids. _____

_____

3. Pericare after each BM. _____

_____

4. Encourage deep breathing exercises and cough q 2 h. _____

_____

5. Reduce environmental stimuli. _____

_____

6. Provide written handout for side effects of medications before discharge. _____

_____

BOX 4-3 APPLICATION OF THE NURSING PROCESS THROUGH THE PLANNING STEP

Step I: Assessment

On 6/11/95 at 5:30 PM, Michelle, a 14-year-old female (DOB 3/2/81), is admitted with a compound multiple fracture of the right tibia and fibula following a mountain bike accident.

ASSESSMENT DATA

Pain/Discomfort

Subjective

Location: R lower leg, as well as general muscle aches and right-sided headache

(Continued)

BOX 4–3 APPLICATION OF THE NURSING PROCESS THROUGH THE PLANNING STEP *(Continued)*

Intensity (1–10): 9
Frequency: Since accident
Quality: Sharp ache (headache dull, throbbing)
Duration: Constant
Radiation: Toes to knee
Precipitating factors: Movement
How relieved: Morphine sulfate in ED
Associated symptoms: Movement, muscle spasms

Objective

Facial grimacing: Yes
Guarding affected area: Yes
Emotional response: Tearful
Narrowed focus: Yes

Step II: Problem Identification

Based on this assessment (and additional data recorded in other sections of the Assessment Tool), using the diagnostic reasoning process and working with Appendix A, you choose the nursing diagnosis label "Pain [acute]," and write the plan of care.

> 6/11/95 6 PM
>
> *Patient Diagnostic Statement:* Pain [acute] related to movement of bone fragments, soft tissue injury/edema, and use of external fixator as evidenced by verbal reports, guarding, muscle tension, narrowed focus, and tachycardia.

Step III: Planning

Goal: Pain-free or controlled.
Outcomes:
> Patient will:

- Verbalize relief of pain within 30 minutes of administration of medication.
- Use relaxation skills to reduce level of pain by 6/12, 9 AM.
- Identify methods that provide relief by 6/12, 4 PM.

Interventions:

- Maintain limb rest of R leg × 24 hours.
- Elevate lower leg with folded blanket.
- Apply ice to area 20 minutes on/20 minutes off, as tolerated × 48 hours.
- Place cradle over foot of bed.
- Document reports and characteristics of pain.
- Medicate with Demerol 75 mg and Phenergan 25 mg IM q 4 h, prn, *or* Vicodin 5 mg po q 4 h, prn.
- Demonstrate/encourage use of progressive relaxation techniques, deep breathing exercises, and visualization.
- Provide alternate comfort measures, position change, backrub. ðð

patient's plan of care, which some nurses refer to as the "care plan." This plan of care is written to:

- ***Provide continuity of care*** from nurse to nurse, from one nursing shift to the next, or from one unit/care setting to another
- ***Enhance communication*** as the written plan becomes a permanent part of the patient record and supplies consistent information for each person who reads it
- ***Assist with determining agency or unit staffing needs,*** setting priorities for the shift work schedule and individual patient assignments
- ***Document the nursing process*** by providing reminders of what needs to be charted and when evaluations should be done
- ***Serve as a teaching tool*** that supports the sharing of nurses' expertise and fosters professional growth as nurses learn what interventions are successful
- ***Coordinate care among disciplines***

The term *health care* is not synonymous with medicine or nursing, but includes many professional disciplines, each of which has its own definite characteristics and independent, but overlapping, functions. Thus, the fields of nursing and medicine are closely related. The relationship includes the exchange of data, the sharing of ideas/thinking, and the development of a plan of care that includes all data pertinent to the individual patient/family/significant others. The same type of relationship also extends to all healthcare disciplines that have contact with the patient.

The implication of this relationship is seen in what is contained in the plan of care, which is more than simply the actions initiated by medical orders (collaborative actions). It also includes a combination of nursing orders (independent actions) and is the written coordination of care given by all health-related disciplines. The nurse becomes the person responsible for seeing to it that all of the different activities are coordinated. This is essential to the delivery of holistic, cost-effective healthcare that promotes optimal patient recovery in a timely manner.

Exercises in "care planning" are assigned to students to increase their mastery of the nursing process and application of related knowledge from other scientific disciplines. The need to identify and prepare for every possible patient problem in a given situation results in the creation of a *case study*, instead of the more abbreviated and succinct plan of care that is usually found in the nursing unit Kardex in most hospitals. However, the length of time and degree of detail required to complete these "case studies" often causes nursing students to develop a negative attitude toward planning care. It is important to keep this activity in perspective, because as a professional nurse, you will need to plan care for your patients on a daily basis. Mastery of the skills of planning care will allow you to complete this activity in a timely fashion as you gain experience.

The plan of care is primarily a communication tool that directs the patient's care. However, newly formulated requirements of outside agencies (for example, JCAHO, Medicare, private insurance companies) stipulate that the nurse is responsible for the planning of patient care and that the plan is to be documented in the patient's record. For these reasons, the plan of care is now

JCAHO—Joint Commission on Accreditation of Healthcare Organizations; surveying body that certifies clinical and organizational performance of an institution following established guidelines.

a permanent part of the patient's record, since it contains the *outline* for the care provided.

DISCHARGE PLANNING

As you plan for the patient's current needs, you must also consider future needs, especially eventual discharge from the healthcare facility. Discharge planning begins when the patient enters the healthcare setting. It is crucial to ensure continuity of care and to take into account the anticipated discharge destination (e.g., home or skilled nursing facility). You are responsible for planning continuity of care between nursing personnel, between services within the care setting, and between the care setting and the community. You may also be responsible for initiating/cooperating in referrals to other community services and providing needed direction for patient/family who are learning to facilitate recovery and promote wellness.

DOCUMENTING THE PLAN OF CARE

The plan of care may be recorded on a single page or in a multiple-page format, such as one page for each diagnostic statement for a particular patient. The page (or pages) may be kept in a folder (Kardex) at the nursing station, in the patient's chart, or at the bedside to communicate and provide direction on a daily basis.

The format for documenting the plan of care is determined by agency policy. Student plans of care (case studies) are individually generated and very detailed. As a practicing professional, you might use a computer with a plan of care data base, standardized care plan forms or CLINICAL PATHWAYS (e.g., Critical Pathway, Care Map, etc.). Whichever you use, the plan of care needs to reflect the basic nursing standards of care, to which personal patient data, nonroutine care, and qualifiers such as time or amount are added, as appropriate.

> CLINICAL PATHWAYS—
> are a type of abbreviated plan of care, providing outcome-based guidelines for goal achievement within a designated length of stay (see Appendix G).

For example:
Measure intake and output [insert frequency]
Increase oral fluids [insert amount and frequency]
Medicate with [insert name of medication, dose, and frequency] for pain
Weigh with bedscale [insert time, frequency]

Some computerized systems for plans of care generate an updated plan at the beginning of each shift. The care provided during the new shift is then recorded directly to the online plan of care throughout that shift. This format serves two purposes: It documents the planning and implementation steps of the nursing process, and it continuously updates the plan of care and the patient's record. Other formats require the nurse to document updates to the plan of care through a notation on the Kardex or in the progress or nursing note.

As previously noted, the plan of care is the visualization of the nursing process. As such, it is preserved as part of the patient's permanent record. Therefore, all entries need to be dated and initialed or signed. Use key words instead of complete sentences and only agency approved abbreviations/symbols (see Appendix G).

PRACTICE ACTIVITY 4-4

DOCUMENTING THE PLAN OF CARE

Instructions: Record the plan of care information from Box 4-3 on pages 82-83 using the following documentation format.

DATE	PATIENT DIAGNOSTIC STATEMENT	GOAL	INTERVENTIONS	OUTCOMES	STATUS

Patient: Donald Age: 46 DOB: 2/4/48 Sex: M   Admission 11/12/94 - 3:40 Dx: Acute Alcoholism/Depression

Date	Patient Diagnostic Statement	Goal	Intervention	Outcomes	Status
11/12	Coping, individual ineffective related to situational crisis of unemployment, personal vulnerability evidenced by reported inability to cope, use of alcohol, insomnia, and diminished problem-solving.	short term: Managing own situation effectively	1. Asseses level of anxiety and Donald's perception of situation	Verbalizes awarenes of sources of anxiety (1000 11/14)	Achieved 11/14 1030 R.S.
			2. Note verbal/nonverbal behaviors of anxiety		
		long term: Expresses sense of self-worth. Maintains sobriety.	3. Look in q 2 hr and PRN		
			4. Encourage verbalization, expression of feelings of denial depression/anger	Demonstrates congruency between feelings/behavior (1000 11/15)	Achieved 11/15 1000 P.D.
			5. Discuss normalcy of these feelings	Demonstrates initial problem-solving skills (1000 11/15)	Achieved 11/15 1000 P.D.
			6. Identify current coping mechanisms	Identifies options and resourses available for assistance (1000 11/16) R. Smith, RN	
			7. Note effectiveness/ need for change		
			8. Discuss/refer to resources: social worker, alcohol counselor, support group, AA		

Figure 4–3. Sample documentation of a plan of care.

For example:
- 8/15 Routine urinary catheter care q (every) shift. RE
- 9/2 NPO (nothing by mouth) after 6 AM, 9/13. PR
- 3/7 Maintain subarachnoid bolt per protocol. MT

Regardless of the format used, the plan of care contains identifying patient data (including medical diagnosis), patient diagnostic statements, goals/outcomes, and interventions, as well as providing space to record the status of the outcomes (i.e., achieved, revised, or deleted) as shown in Figure 4–3. After reviewing the figure, take a moment to complete Practice Activity 4–4.

VALIDATING THE PLAN OF CARE

Before the plan of care is implemented, it should be reviewed to ensure that:
- It is based on accepted nursing practice reflecting knowledge of scientific principles, nursing standards of care, and agency policies.

PRACTICE ACTIVITY 4-5

PLANNING

Desired Outcome and Patient Criteria: The Patient will:

TIME OUT! The desired outcome must meet criteria to be accurate. The outcome must be specific, realistic, measurable, and include a time frame for completion. Does the action verb describe the patient's behavior to be evaluated? Can the outcome be used in the evaluation step of the nursing process to measure the patient's response to the nursing interventions listed below?

Interventions	Rationale for Selected Intervention and References

EVALUATION

TIME OUT! Do your interventions assist in achieving the desired outcome? Do your interventions address further monitoring of the patient's response to your interventions and to the achievement of the desired outcome? Are qualifiers: **when, how, amount, time,** and **frequency** used? Is the focus of the action's verb on the nurse's actions and not on the patient? Do your rationales provide sufficient reason and directions?

What was your patient's response to the interventions?

Was the desired outcome achieved? ☐ Yes ☐ No   If no, what revisions to either the desired outcome or interventions would you make?

DOCUMENTATION

Documentation Focus: Now that you have completed the evaluation, the next step is to document your care and the patient's response. Use the areas below to enter your progress note information.

Reassessment Data:

Interventions Implemented:

Patient's Response:

INSTRUCTOR'S COMMENTS:

- It provides for the safety of the patient by ensuring that the care provided will do no harm.
- The patient diagnostic statements are supported by the patient data.
- The goals and outcomes are measurable/observable and can be achieved.
- The interventions can benefit the patient/significant others in a predictable way to achieve the identified outcomes and are arranged in a logical sequence.
- It demonstrates individualized patient care by including the concerns of the patient and significant others as well as their physical and psychosocial needs and capabilities.

PROFESSIONAL CONCERNS RELATED TO THE PLAN OF CARE

Professional concerns associated with the identification of patient problems/needs in the construction of the plan of care are:

- What is the nurse's responsibility once a nursing diagnosis is made if the patient is discharged from care before all short-term outcomes are met or problems are resolved?
- Who is responsible for follow-through in providing and evaluating care once the patient has been discharged?
- Who is responsible for monitoring patient progress toward long-term outcomes?
- Should this information be shared with the patient's admitting/primary physician or office nurse?
- Is the nurse who has made a nursing diagnosis responsible for follow-through to its resolution?

Nationally, these questions are unresolved, and patient outcomes may remain unmet. Ethically, it is up to the nursing community and the healthcare industry to formulate policies that will promote optimal patient recovery and health maintenance. As a healthcare professional, you need to consider these issues because they will affect the care you provide and the way you develop the plan of care for your patient.

PUTTING IT ALL TOGETHER

Practice Activity 4–5 presents the back page of the interactive plan of care worksheet described and used in Chapter 3. The information included on the worksheet and in the TIME OUT sections should give you another view of the steps of the nursing process described in this chapter. Return to Practice Activity 3–3 at the end of Chapter 3 and see what portion of the information you can include based on the subjective and objective data of your patient Robert, who, as you remember, was diagnosed with Activity Intolerance. What desired outcome would you identify for Robert? The TIME OUT sections will give you evaluation criteria to ensure Robert's outcome statement is correctly written. Once again, the TIME OUT sections give you guidance in correctly writing your nursing interventions.

BOX 4–4   MEASUREMENT CRITERIA FOR ANA STANDARD III AND IV

ANA Standard III: Outcome Identification: The nurse identifies expected outcomes individualized to the client.

1. Outcomes are derived from the diagnoses.
2. Outcomes are documented as measurable goals.
3. Outcomes are mutually formulated with the client and healthcare providers, when possible.
4. Outcomes are realistic in relation to the client's present and potential capabilities.
5. Outcomes are attainable in relation to resources available to the client.
6. Outcomes include a time estimate for attainment.
7. Outcomes provide direction for continuity of care.

ANA Standard IV: Planning: The nurse develops a plan of care that prescribes interventions to attain expected outcomes.

1. The plan is individualized to the client's condition or needs.
2. The plan is developed with the client, significant other(s), and health-care providers, when appropriate.
3. The plan reflects current nursing practice.
4. The plan is documented.
5. The plan provides for continuity of care.

SUMMARY

Healthcare providers have a responsibility to plan care with the patient and family whether the desired outcome is an optimal state of wellness or a dignified death. Planning care by setting goals, determining outcomes, and choosing appropriate interventions are essential to the delivery of quality nursing care. These nursing activities comprise the Planning step of the Nursing Process, and are documented in the plan of care for a particular patient. As a part of the patient's permanent record, the plan of care not only provides a means for the nurse who is actively caring for the patient to be aware of the problems (nursing diagnoses), goals, and actions to be taken, but it also substantiates the plan of care for third-party payors, accreditation, and legal needs.

Now, return to the third and fourth standards of the ANA Standard of Clinical Nursing Practice and review the measurement criteria necessary to achieve and ensure compliance with each standard. The knowledge and skill required to meet the criteria listed in Box 4–4 were described in this chapter.

The next chapter provides information on the fourth step of the nursing process, IMPLEMENTATION. You will have an opportunity to see how the plan of care can be implemented. In order to achieve the desired outcomes, you will learn what mechanisms help to prioritize the nursing interventions that were selected during the Planning step. Finally, you will practice effective communication methods to help ensure the required continuity of care described in the patient plan of care.

WORK PAGE: Chapter Four

1. List three reasons why the plan of care is important:

    a. _____

    b. _____

    c. _____

2. Briefly explain why setting priorities is necessary: _____

_____

_____

3. What is the difference between a goal and an outcome? _____

_____

_____

_____

4. Identify five important components of patient outcomes:

    a. _____

    b. _____

    c. _____

    d. _____

    e. _____

5. List four types of information that nursing interventions need to contain:

    a. _____

    b. _____

    c. _____

    d. _____

6. Explain the difference between a measurable and a nonmeasurable verb and give an example of

    each: _____

_____

_____

7. When does discharge planning begin? _____

_____

8. How is the plan of care documented? _____

_____

9. Identify two additional problems facing Michelle; then set a goal with one outcome and two interventions for each problem.

Vignette: Michelle, the 14-year-old female with compound fractures of the right lower leg, has other problems in addition to Pain [acute], as previously discussed. Her wound was contaminated by dirt and she had significant blood loss before paramedics arrived. Although the wound was flushed with sterile saline and antibiotic solution before being packed and dressed, a cast was not applied because of tissue swelling and concerns about the wound and bone. Instead, an external fixation device (a metal frame with pins extending through the skin and bone) is currently being used for immobilization of the tibia and fibula. The device is heavy and awkward for Michelle to move without causing increased pain, and she is to remain on bedrest for 24 hours. In addition, IV antibiotics are to be administered every 4 hours.

a. Problem: _____

_____

Goal: _____

Outcome: _____

Interventions:

1. _____

2. _____

b. Problem: _____

_____

Goal: _____

Outcome: _____

Interventions:

1. _____

2. _____

BIBLIOGRAPHY

Bulechek, G.M., & McCloskey, J.C. (1989). *Nursing interventions: Treatments for Potential Diagnoses.* In Carrol-Johnson, R.M. (Ed.), Proceedings of Eighth Conference, NANDA. Philadelphia: J.B. Lippincott.

Bulechek, G.M., & McCloskey, J.C. (1992). *Nursing Interventions: Essential Nursing Treatments* (2nd ed.). Philadelphia: W.B. Saunders.

Kalish, R. (1983). *The Psychology of Human Behavior* (5th ed.). Monterey, CA: Brooks/Cole.

Maslow, A.H. (1970). *Motivation and Personality* (2nd ed.). New York: Harper & Row.

McCloskey, J.C., & Bulechek, G.M. (Eds.). (1992). *Nursing Interventions Classification (NIC).* St. Louis, MO: Mosby—Year Book.

Snyder, M. (1985). *Independent Nursing Interventions.* New York: Wiley.

Snyder, M. (1992). *Independent Nursing Interventions* (2nd ed.). Albany, NY: Delmar.

SUGGESTED READING

Carpenito, L.J. (1991). *Nursing Care Plans and Documentation.* Philadelphia: J.B. Lippincott.

Cox, H., et al. (1993). *Clinical Applications of Nursing Diagnosis: Adult Health, Child Health, Women's Health, Mental Health, and Home Health* (2nd ed.). Philadelphia: F.A. Davis.

Craft, M.J., & Denehy, J.A. (1990). *Nursing Interventions for Infants and Children.* Philadelphia: W.B. Saunders.

Doenges, M.E., & Moorhouse, M.F. (1993). *Nurse's Pocket Guide: Nursing Diagnoses With Interventions* (4th ed.). Philadelphia: F.A. Davis.

Doenges, M.E., Moorhouse, M.F., & Geissler, A.C. (1993). *Nursing Care Plans: Guidelines for Planning and Documenting Patient Care* (3rd ed.). Philadelphia: F.A. Davis.

Holloway, N.M. (1993). *Medical-Surgical Care Planning* (2nd ed.). Springhouse, PA: Springhouse.

Leuner, J.D., Manton, A.K., Kelliher, D.B., Sullivan, S.P., & Doherty, M. (1990). *Mastering the Nursing Process: A Case Study Approach.* Philadelphia: F.A. Davis.

Maas, M., Buckwalter, K.C., & Hardy, M. (1991). *Nursing Diagnosis and Interventions for the Elderly.* Menlo Park, CA: Addison-Wesley.

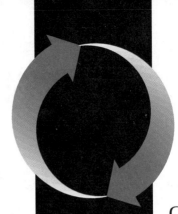

CHAPTER 5

The Implementation Step: Putting the Plan of Care into Action

---

- ■ **Identifying Caregiving Priorities**
- ■ **Delivering Nursing Care**
- ■ **Ongoing Data Collection**
     Documentation
     Verbal Communication with the Healthcare Team
- ■ **Summary**

ANA Standard 5: Implementation: The nurse implements the interventions identified in the plan of care.

At this point of the nursing process, you are ready to perform the interventions and activities recorded in the patient's plan of care. In order to IMPLE-MENT this plan in a timely and cost-effective manner, you first identify the priorities for providing patient care. Then as care is provided, you monitor and document the patient's response to each of the interventions and communicate this information to other healthcare providers as appropriate. Then, using the data, you evaluate and revise the plan of care in the following step of the nursing process (see Chapter 6).

IMPLEMENT/IMPLEMENTA-TION—fourth step of nursing process in which the plan of care is put into action; performing identified interventions/activities.

95

PRACTICE ACTIVITY 5–1

SETTING YOUR WORK SCHEDULE FOR IMPLEMENTING THE PLAN OF CARE

Vignette: Michelle incurred a compound fracture of the right lower leg 2 days ago. In reviewing the plan of care, you take note of the following:

- Assist with bed bath
- Calculate I & O every 8 hours (2 PM)
- Change dressing twice a day and prn (9 AM, 9 PM)
- Assess vital signs every 4 hours (8 AM, 12 noon)
- Monitor circulation/nerve function R lower leg every hour x 24 hours, then every 4 hours and prn.
- IV medications 8 AM, 2 PM
- Up in chair with meals (7:30 AM, 12 noon)
- Walk in halls three times a day after instructed in crutch walking

1. Organize the above interventions and activities on the worksheet below:

Worksheet

Pt.	7	8	9	10	11	12	1	2	3	Comments

2. During nursing rounds, just after the change-of-shift report on 3/13, you find Michelle is crying and she reports sudden throbbing pain in her right lower leg. How will this affect your

   work plan? _____

   _____

IDENTIFYING CAREGIVING PRIORITIES

Regardless of how well a plan of care has been constructed, it cannot predict everything that will occur with a particular patient on a daily basis. Your individual knowledge base, expertise, and recognition of agency routines allows you to exhibit the flexibility necessary to adapt to the changing needs of the patient. While listening closely to the change-of-shift report, you will get the first clues about where to begin. On a worksheet such as the one shown in Figure 5–1 or a form supplied by the agency, you record specific information, in-

Pt.	7	8	9	10	11	12	1	2	3	Comments
Rbt		Vital signs Chair	Med	Bed bath	IV	V.S. Chair	Med	I & O		

Figure 5–1. Sample worksheet for the 7:00 AM to 3:00 PM shift. While listening to the change-of-shift report, you review the plan of care and begin to plan how you will implement specific interventions. You notice that Robert is to eat meals sitting up in a chair; therefore, he should be helped out of bed before the meal trays arrive on the unit. You identify times for medications, time for expected change of the IV bottle, and the routine time for calculating the intake and output for the shift. In addition, you are aware that Robert's family usually visits at lunch time, so you schedule hygiene needs appropriately while allowing Robert rest periods between activities.

terventions, or activities that are sequential or time related. Also, you review the plan of care for outcomes that are to be evaluated during the shift and for routine procedures/treatments and medication administration. Complete Practie Activity 5–1 at this time.

After completion of the shift report, performing a baseline assessment of each patient can provide clues about general physical status, equipment/supply needs, and safety concerns (e.g., patency of invasive lines [catheters/tubes] and intravenous [IV] flow rate). At this time you may recognize a change in the significance or severity of a patient problem which could affect the plan of care.

> **For example:** Robert, who is being treated for pneumonia, appears dyspneic at 7:30 AM. You will need to do a more thorough focused assessment now to determine his immediate needs. This could include obtaining arterial blood gases (ABGs) and restarting supplemental oxygen. In addition, you may decide against getting Robert up in a chair to eat his breakfast. Thus, interventions previously identified are not appropriate at this time, and new or alternate interventions are needed.

This is also the time to review the plan of care with the patient/significant other to schedule activities and verify the patient's responsibilities.

> **For example:** Donald, admitted 48 hours ago for depression and alcohol withdrawal, displays coarse tremors of his hands and an unsteady gait and requires assistance with self-care. It is 7:30 AM and breakfast trays have just arrived. Donald is required to attend the Community Meeting at 8:15 AM before proceeding to individually prescribed activities. Donald is ambivalent about his morning care, but in reviewing the scheduled activities, he decides he will postpone his shower until his 10:30 AM break.

Finally, legal and ethical concerns related to the interventions need to be considered. The wishes of the patient and family/significant others regarding what is being done need to be discussed and respected.

> **For example:** Robert has decided that if he should suffer respiratory failure, he is not to be placed on a mechanical ventilator. This does not

PRACTICE ACTIVITY 5–2

LEGAL AND ETHICAL CONCERNS OF CARE

As noted, Robert had completed a form directing healthcare providers to withhold advanced life-support measures including the use of a mechanical ventilator.

1. Have you and your family members completed advance directives stating specific healthcare

   desires? _____

   If not, why: _____

   _____

2. As a nurse, how do you feel about adhering to advance directives as stipulated by an elderly

   patient? _____

   _____

   for a premature infant as stipulated by the parents? _____

   _____

3. Review the Code for Nurses (see Appendix D) and choose two principles you believe may address your responsibility to patient's/guardian's in regard to their decisions limiting care.

   _____

   _____

negate the need for intervention when you notice that he is developing problems. You still need to act promptly to prevent or limit further deterioration. Therefore, in addition to providing oxygen and assessing breath sounds and airway patency, you elevate the head of Robert's bed, encourage Robert to deep-breathe and cough regularly, and notify other healthcare providers (e.g., physician and respiratory therapist) as appropriate, as well as the identified family member or contact person.

Take a few minutes to consider the legal and ethical concerns of Robert's decision and work through Practice Activity 5–2 before continuing with the next section.

DELIVERING NURSING CARE

Interventions may be composed of many activities ranging from simple tasks to complex procedures. These activities may require direct "hands-on" care (such as a complete bed bath) or may merely require assisting a patient by setting up a basin of water and washing his back. Other frequent activities include instructing a patient and/or significant other regarding the management of care and then supervising these efforts. The patient and/or significant others may need to be counseled regarding psychosocial concerns, treatment regimens, or alternative ways to manage healthcare needs. Throughout these activities, you also monitor the patient and such resources as diagnostic studies and/or progress reports from other healthcare providers for changes in health status/development of complications.

Before implementing the interventions listed in the plan of care, you need to be sure that you:

- *Understand the reason for doing the intervention, its expected effect, and any potential hazards that can occur.* Without this knowledge, the nurse cannot be sure that the intervention will be beneficial. In addition, it will be difficult to determine if the desired effect is being achieved or if adaptations are required to provide for specific patient needs/safety concerns.

    For example: You realize that an ABG study will provide information about Robert's current oxygenation status/needs, and also that he requires supplemental oxygen to increase his oxygen level. That means you will implement these interventions in a slightly different sequence; that is, the diagnostic study (ABG) should be obtained *before* the supplemental oxygen is begun, so that test results are not affected by the additional oxygen.

- *Provide an environment or milieu conducive to carrying out the planned interventions.* What is happening in the patient's environment is known to affect the person's physical and psychological self (e.g., noise, temperature, activities).

    For example: Exposing Robert for a bed bath when the room is cold can cause him physical discomfort, as well as affect his psychological response. Michelle has difficulty focusing on your instructions for administering medications when the volume of her roommate's TV is turned up and visitors are talking loudly.

- *Consider which interventions can be combined so you can accomplish the activities within your time constraints.* In some cases, shortcuts may be chosen or activities combined as long as consideration is given to the successful accomplishment of the outcome.

    For example: While administering Valium to Donald at 8:00 AM, you can review the drug's actions, side-effects, and adverse reactions. Or while assisting Sally with her sitz bath, you may choose to discuss her concerns about caring for herself and the new babies once she is discharged.

As noted in Box 5–1, one "simple" intervention such as providing a bedpan for a patient actually encompasses multiple nursing activities that, when listed individually, may appear to take considerable time and energy to perform. However, by carefully prioritizing interventions and sequencing related activities you can accomplish these tasks quickly.

BOX 5-1   THE TRUTH ABOUT BEDPANS

Even the simplest of nursing tasks is really a complex series of actions and judgments, requiring professional knowledge and experience in order to provide optimal patient care. Read through the short article reprinted below.* You will be surprised to see just how complicated supplying a patient with a bedpan can be.

There are many nursing activities interwoven in the "simple" act of providing a bedpan. As a nurse, you assess the patient's:

> Level of consciousness and mood, including self-image while dependent with these bodily functions.
> Skin color, temperature, and suppleness.
> Respiratory pattern and rate, breath sounds, and dyspnea with or without activity.
> Comfort level with voiding or with stool.
> Range of motion, strength, and any pain with movement.
> Urine for color, amount, odor, and by-products such as mucus or blood.
> Stool for color, consistency, amount, and by-products such as mucus, undigested food, or blood.

You also determine:

> If urine assessment relates to medications (Lasix, Pyridium, aminoglycosides), fluid intake, disease process (diabetes, dehydration, renal failure), or infection.
> If stool assessment relates to medication (antibiotics, barium enema, narcotics), food or fluid intake, disease process (cholelithiasis, Crohn's disease, bleeding ulcers), infection, activity or inactivity.
> If assessment demands any action and whether the doctor needs to be notified.

You then go on to teach:

> Symptoms to watch for, comfort measures, and ways to maintain or achieve normal functioning.
> Disease process and how it affects the individual.

On top of all that you:

> Promote self-esteem by using proper technique, including disposal of waste material.
> Obtain necessary specimens using correct procedure and send to lab.
> Make sure patient is clean and dry to promote good skin integrity.
> Model good handwashing technique upon completion.

* "The Truth about Bedpans" by Karen Tolin, RN, Joplin, MO, printed by *RN Magazine*.

ONGOING DATA COLLECTION

Once you have formulated the plan of care and put it into action, monitor the patient to collect additional data. As you talk to the patient, note changes in tone of voice and expression, or when providing a back rub, be aware of such abnormalities as a reddened area on the coccyx. All of these data need to be noted, and their meaning validated. This information will be used to make decisions regarding the need for new goals, outcomes, interventions, and reprioritizing the plan of care during the evaluation process.

Documentation

It is legally required that all healthcare settings document nursing observations, the care provided, and the patient's response. This record serves as a communication tool and a resource to aid in determining the effectiveness of care and to assist in setting priorities for ongoing care. In order to simplify record-keeping and to promote timely and accurate charting, many agencies use flow sheets to document routine activities, monitoring, and patient care (Fig. 5–2). Flow sheets reduce the need to write detailed progress notes. Instead, only variations from the recorded baseline and any exceptions requiring more explanation are written in the progress note. Additional discussion about documentation and the use of progress notes will be presented in Chapter 7.

Verbal Communication with the Healthcare Team

In addition to the written record, patient information is shared verbally with other healthcare providers. Whether reporting to another nurse, reviewing with a physician, or discussing with other resources (e.g., social worker, dietitian, or physical therapist), the manner in which information is conveyed, as well as the content itself, can affect the way in which this information is heard. This, in turn, can have an impact on the quality of the health care provided. For this reason, it is important to avoid judgmental language, tone of voice, or body language. Presenting information in an objective and accurate manner reduces the likelihood of being misunderstood or of negatively influencing the patient's care.

> **For example:** When Sally talked to the nurse, expressing concern about going home, the nurse reported this information to the oncoming shift personnel and to the doctor by saying: "I think Sally is trying to manipulate us. She says she's not ready to go home, and she thinks if she 'acts weak,' she won't have to leave the hospital."

After listening to this judgmental report, the oncoming nurse's response might be one of defensiveness and the nurse might be inclined to *show* Sally that she is indeed ready to go home. The nurse may also subconsciously stop listening and is likely to be less receptive to what Sally *is* saying. Contrast the above example with the one which appears below.

> **For example:** If the nurse reports: "Sally has expressed concern about her ability to manage at home. She was weak when we got her up this morning, requiring assistance with walking. Then she spent the afternoon talking on the telephone, at one point ignoring the cries of Baby B until I responded to the room. We need information about her situation at home and her need for assistance with newborn care of twins."

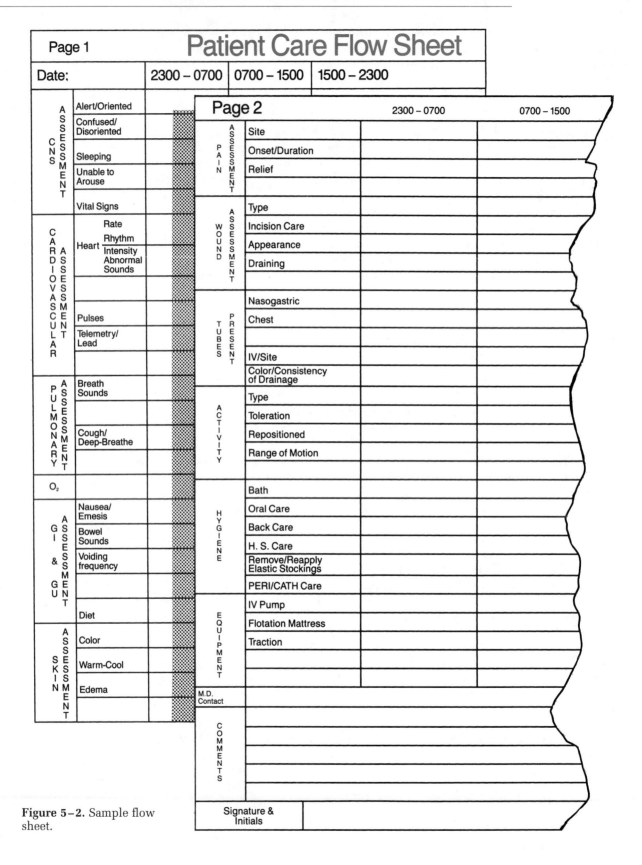

Figure 5–2. Sample flow sheet.

In this report, the nurse expresses a problem in terms that challenge colleagues to find a solution. This problem is approached with an open mind, as additional data are gathered and appropriate resources are identified. Maintaining an open mind and actively problem-solving provides opportunities for creating solutions instead of additional problems, thus promoting a positive patient/nurse experience.

The primary format for communicating the patient's current situation and needs is the nursing change-of-shift report. This type of report may be done either in person or via tape recorder. As time for this activity is usually limited, it is necessary to be brief and organized while still providing pertinent data. After supplying basic patient data (e.g., room number, name, age, diagnosis, and physician), reporting may be done "by exception." This means that only occurrences that are out of the ordinary are reported. You report:

- *Abnormalities/changes in assessment findings*
  "Robert became short of breath during AM rounds and required supplemental oxygen at 2 L/min by nasal cannula." Or "Michelle's right lower leg edema is resolving."
- *Diagnostic procedures and results*
  "Robert's oxygen saturation is 92 percent on 2 liters of oxygen; chest x-ray report is pending."
- *Variations from usual routine*
  "Robert was not out of bed this AM but was up for lunch and tolerated sitting up in a chair for 45 mintues without difficulty."
- *Activities not completed on your shift*
  "The crutches are in Michelle's room, a physical therapist will return at 4 PM to instruct her in their use; then we can begin getting her out of bed."
- *Status of invasive treatments*
  "Sally's IV of lactated Ringer's with 2 amps of Pitocin is infusing in the left forearm at 60 mL/hr with 300 mL remaining."
- *Additions or changes to the plan of care* (this includes evaluation of outcomes and the status of patient problems) "Robert's Airway Clearance problem has recurred requiring aggressive pulmonary toilet every 2 hours and use of incentive spirometer."

Change-of-shift reports may include nursing rounds, with each patient being visited by the offgoing and oncoming nurse together. Nursing rounds are beneficial in verifying the status of invasive treatments, appearance of wounds/dressings, and the current condition of the patient (e.g., degree of jaundice, level of coolness of an extremity, etc.). It is imperative to maintain the confidentiality of patient information, and usually it is preferable to review the change-of-shift information before going to the patient's bedside.

Patient confidentiality is an ethical/moral concern that must be respected by each professional at all times. These concerns are extended to conversations at the nursing station, on the telephone, or wherever patient information is discussed. This includes refraining from discussions with those not directly involved in the patient's care (e.g., staff on other units, your own family, friends and acquaintances of the patient).

Before concluding this chapter, take a moment to complete Practice Activity 5–3.

PRACTICE ACTIVITY 5-3

COMMUNICATING NURSING INFORMATION TO OTHER CAREGIVERS

Work through the questions below.

1. Two methods of communicating your observations about patient care and activities to other nurses are by:

a. _____

b. _____

2. Discuss the benefits of nursing rounds: _____

_____

3. Underline the information listed below that you would include in your change-of-shift report:

Sally   Ate well   Age 30   Dr. Jefferson
Weak and unsteady while up in hall
Episiotomy reddened, slight edema, no drainage second day postpartum
Scheduled for discharge tomorrow
Received oral pain medication at 11 AM with reported relief
Does not want to go home
Sister in to visit at lunchtime
Coordination for home care services in progress with the Discharge Planner
Spent afternoon talking on phone
Has not named Baby B and at times has ignored infant cues

4. The wife of a prominent local politician is admitted for treatment of alcoholism. You could discuss her admission and course of therapy with which of the following people?

_____ attending/primary physician
_____ the nursing supervisor
_____ a pediatric nurse (her best friend)
_____ your husband
_____ the patient's son
_____ an interested newspaper reporter
_____ other nurses on your unit

SUMMARY

In putting the plan of care into action and providing effective patient care, you review resources to determine priorities, consulting with and considering the desires of the patient during this Implementation step of the nursing process. You identify who is responsible for the actions to be taken and set realistic timeframes for carrying out actions. Changes in the patient's needs must be continually monitored because patient care takes place in a dynamic environment. The relevance of new data collected in each interaction with the patient is determined according to what is already known. This newly gathered information is documented and shared with other healthcare providers as appropriate. Throughout these activities, flexibility is important to allow for changed circumstances, interruptions, and so forth.

Before we begin the next chapter, let us return to the fifth standard of the ANA Standard of Clinical Nursing Practice and review the measurement criteria necessary to achieve and ensure compliance with the standard. The knowledge and skill required to meet the criteria listed in Box 5–2 were described in this chapter on the IMPLEMENTATION step of the nursing process.

Chapter 6 will help you see how continuous evaluation of nursing actions helps you determine whether or not the interventions are leading to achievement of the desired outcomes. In addition, evaluation of patient plans of care serves as a mechanism for review of the care provided on a unit or within an agency. This review process addresses professional issues of overall quality of care and also provides a means by which outside agencies can evaluate the institution.

WORK PAGE: Chapter Five

1. Identify three activities involved in implementing the plan of care:

   a. _____

   b. _____

   c. _____

2. Discuss the importance of understanding the expected effect and potential hazards of the interventions you will implement: _____

   _____

3. Explain the purpose for ongoing data collection throughout the Implementation step of the nursing process: _____

   _____

4. List two reasons why documentation of the care provided is important:

   a. _____

   b. _____

5. Name three activities you might use to carry out interventions for planned patient care:

   a. _____   b. _____   c. _____

6. What is the advantage of reporting "by exception?" _____

   _____

7. When and where is patient confidentiality important? _____

   _____

8. Flexibility in providing patient care is important because: _____

   _____

9.

Vignette: Robert signed advanced directives asking that no extraordinary means (e.g., intubation and mechanical ventilation) be used to prolong his life. When his condition changed, his daughter was notified as required. While visiting with her father, she is surprised to learn of his decision. She is very upset and a confrontation develops. Robert tells her "it is none of your business" and refuses to enter into further conversation.

a. What can you do now? _____

_____

BIBLIOGRAPHY

Coleman, S., & Henneman, E.A. (1991). Comprehensive patient care and documentation through unit-based nursing rounds. *Clinical Nurse Specialist, 5*(2), 117–120.

Concern for Dying. (1991). *Advance Directive Protocols and the Patient Self-Determination Act.* New York: Author.

Daniels, N. (1985). *Just Health Care.* Cambridge University Press. Cambridge, MA.

Daniels, N. (1988). *Am I My Parent's Keeper: An Essay on Justice Between the Young and the Old.* New York: Oxford.

Doenges, M.E., & Moorhouse, M.F. (1993). *Nurses's Pocket Guide: Nursing Diagnoses with Interventions* (4th ed.). Philadelphia: F.A. Davis.

McCloskey, J.C., & Grace, H.L. (Eds.). (1994). *Current Issues in Nursing.* St. Louis, MO: C.V. Mosby.

Monahan, M.L., Bacha, H., Pheips, C., & Whatley, H. (1988). Change of shift report: A time for communication with patients. *Nursing Management, 19*(2), 80.

Reiley, P.J., & Stengrevics, S.S. (1989). Change of shift report: Put it in writing! *Nursing Management, 20*(9), 54–56.

White, G.B. (1992). *Ethical Dilemmas in Contemporary Nursing Practice.* Washington, DC: American Nurses Publishing.

Wolf, Z.R. (1989). Learning the professional jargon of nursing during change of shift report. *Holistic Nursing Practice, 4*(1), 78–83.

Veins, D.C. (1989). A history of nursing's code of ethics. *Nursing Outlook, 37*(1), 43–49.

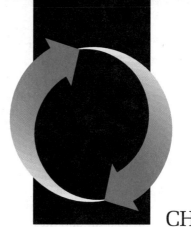

CHAPTER 6

The Evaluation Step: Determining Whether Desired Outcomes Have Been Met

---

- ■ **Reassessment**
- ■ **Modification of the Plan of Care**
- ■ **Termination of Services**
- ■ **Enhancing Delivery of Quality Care**
- ■ **Summary**

ANA Standard 6: Evaluation: The nurse evaluates the client's progress toward attainment of outcomes.

EVALUATION—final step of the nursing process. A continuous process essential to assuring the quality and appropriateness of the care provided that is done by reviewing patient responses to determine effectiveness of the plan of care in meeting patient needs.

The final step of the nursing process is evaluating the patient's response to the care delivered to make sure the desired outcomes developed in the Planning step and documented in the plan of care have been achieved. EVALUATION, which is an ongoing process, is necessary for determining how well the plan of care is working. As the patient's condition changes, information is added to the patient data base, requiring revision and updating of the plan of care, which is an essential component of the Evaluation step.

Although the process of evaluation may seem similar to the activity of as-

109

sessment, there are important differences. Instead of identifying the patient's general status and problems/needs, the evaluation focuses on the *appropriateness* of the care provided and the patient's progress or lack of progress toward the desired outcomes. Evaluation is an interactive, continuous process. As each nursing action is performed, the patient's response is noted and *evaluated* in relation to the identified outcomes. Then, based on the patient's response, appropriate revisions of nursing interventions and/or patient outcomes may be necessary.

Although it is frequently viewed simplistically as a pass or fail judgment, evaluation should actually be seen as a constructive opportunity to provide positive feedback to both the patient and caregivers for their efforts, and encouragement to continue to strive for a higher level of functioning or wellness. It is an opportunity for problem solving and personal growth. The Evaluation step has three components: Reassessment, Modification of the plan of care, and finally, Termination of services. The first two components form a continuous loop of recurring assessment and reaction, which eventually leads to the third component. This "termination of services" may sound rather abrupt, but this final part of the evaluation step is in reality the next step for the patient in looking toward the future and "moving on." Termination in part includes completion of discharge planning and addresses those patient nursing diagnoses or patient needs that were not fully attained during the hospitalization. Further description of this part of the evaluation step is presented later in this chapter.

REASSESSMENT

Reassessment is a constant "monitoring" of the patient's status that looks at the patient's response to nursing interventions and progress toward attaining the desired outcome. This evaluation process is ongoing; it does not just occur when an outcome is to be reviewed or a determination of the patient's readiness for discharge is to be made. Data collected as the plan of care was implemented in step 4 of the nursing process are now evaluated or reassessed. Evaluation of the data determines:

- *The appropriateness of the nursing actions*

  For example: Robert's dyspnea has resolved with the provision of oxygen and attention to pulmonary toilet (i.e., periodic deep breathing exercises, effective cough, position changes, and use of the incentive spirometer).

- *The need to revise the interventions*

  For example: Robert was kept in bed for breakfast but should be able to be out of bed for lunch. Or while you were assisting Michelle to walk the length of the hall, you noted that she is unsteady on her crutches and will initially require the assistance of two individuals to provide for patient and employee safety.

- *The development of new patient problems/needs*

  For example: Sally is scheduled for discharge tomorrow. Her current weakness and lack of attention to her infant's cues raise concerns about her current coping abilities and the potential for parenting/attachment problems as well as issues of self-care.

- *The need for referral to other resources*

  For example: Sally's physician is notified of your observations, and possible solutions are discussed. A family meeting may be requested, to clarify roles/responsibilities and availability of assistance. The home health nurse is to be contacted to arrange self-care and home-maker assistance and to supervise Sally's situation after discharge. Referrals to community support groups (such as Mothers of Twins) may be made to provide additional assistance and problem-solving options.

- *The need to rearrange priorities to meet the changing demands of care*

  For example: You had planned to get Robert up in the chair for breakfast, but the focused assessment revealed a change in his respiratory status requiring new interventions and revision of the plan. Or external factors may occur such as the emergency department calls to say they have a new patient requiring admission. You need to review and reschedule the activities planned for Robert in order to accommodate these additional and unplanned responsibilities.

While evaluating the patient's response to care, you also note progress toward the specified outcomes. In addition, as each outcome has an identified timeframe, achievement of the outcomes is periodically reviewed. You must now determine whether the outcomes have been met completely, partially, or not at all; and whether or not the plan of care needs to be revised. Outcome(s) may be evaluated by:

- *Direct observation*

  For example: Did the patient ambulate the length of the hall without developing dyspnea? Did the patient demonstrate proper technique for the administration of insulin? Is the patient free of skin breakdown?

- *Patient interview*

  For example: Does the patient report decreased level of pain after administration of oral pain medication? Can the patient list available community resources? Is the patient able to verbalize the signs/symptoms that require medical evaluation or follow-up?

- *Review of records:* (e.g., progress notes, flow sheets, medication record)

  For example: Has the patient's temperature remained within normal range? Are the intake and output balanced? Has the patient gained weight? Has a laxative been required for constipation?

An important aspect of this process is the involvement of the patient. How does the patient believe she or he is doing? Inclusion of the patient's point of view can provide important insights that will provide additional data for evaluating and revising the plan of care.

If the outcomes were completely met, ask yourself the following questions: "Which interventions can be terminated?" "How easily were the outcomes achieved?" "Can timelines be shortened?" To determine why an outcome was not met, questions such as those noted in Box 6–1 may help to provide clarification.

BOX 6-1   UNMET OUTCOMES—QUESTIONS TO ASK

If the outcomes have not been met completely, questions to be considered are:

- Were the outcomes realistic and appropriate?
- Was the patient involved in setting the outcomes?
- Does the patient believe the outcomes were important?
- Does the patient know why the outcomes have not been met?
- Have all the interventions that were identified been carried out and in the timeframe specified?
  If not, why not? Were they too vague or misinterpreted?
- What variables may have affected achievement of the outcomes?
- Were new problems/adverse patient responses detected early enough to make appropriate changes in the plan of care?

In addition, you review the orders and progress notes of all healthcare providers and identify factors that helped or hindered achievement of outcomes. The findings are then documented on the plan of care and/or progress notes as appropriate and shared with the patient.

MODIFICATION OF THE PLAN OF CARE

When you have completed evaluating the outcomes and the plan of care, you may find the patient's condition has changed in a direction that was or was not anticipated regardless of your nursing interventions and the patient's desire to achieve the stated outcomes. At this point, a change in treatment approach is indicated and the plan of care must be modified to reflect these changes.

As basic physiologic needs such as air, water, food, and safety are met, nursing care can progress to such higher-level concerns as self-esteem. Alternatively, when dealing with higher-level needs they may be put "on hold," while those associated with *newly* emerging basic needs are addressed. At any time, the nurse may identify or activate additional patient diagnostic statements, goals, and/or desired outcomes and corresponding interventions. An earlier chapter discussed the difficulty dealing with more than three to five patient problems at one time. The actual number varies from patient to patient and the complexity of the nursing diagnoses present, but the point is, there may simply be too many patient needs to address in the initial plan of care. Priority setting is required when this situation exists, with progression to higher-level needs as the patient's condition permits.

When the desired outcomes are evaluated and found to be unmet, the reasons need to be identified and documented, and the outcomes then revised or new ones written. When revising patient outcomes, keep in mind that they may simply need to be restated, or their timeframes lengthened so that the patient can successfully achieve them.

> **For example:** When Donald was first admitted for acute alcoholism and depression, the initial concerns focused on issues of patient safety/poten-

tial for injury, changes in sensory interpretation, anxiety, and general nutrition. When Donald completed his initial withdrawal from alcohol and his physical condition stabilized, nursing attention became focused on previously identified problems concerning individual coping and role performance.

As the plan of care is modified, remember to address the changing needs of the patient/significant others, the changes in the patient's health status, environment, and therapeutic regimen. To assist in this process, a patient care conference may be scheduled or a consultation with a colleague or other resource people with special knowledge may be necessary to provide additional insight and to problem-solve solutions.

Practice Activity 6–1 (see page 116) provides an opportunity to review and evaluate the plan of care for Michelle. Read the narrative accompanying Michelle's plan of care and follow the directions for evaluating whether Michelle had attained the stated outcomes. Write your evaluations in the STATUS column of the plan of care. Once you have completed Practice Activity 6–1, turn to Practice Activity 6–2 (see page 116) and add your modifications to Michelle's plan of care in the provided space.

TERMINATION OF SERVICES

When the desired outcomes have been achieved and the broader goals met, termination of care is planned. You now focus on how the patient will manage on his or her own. While termination of care occurs when all goals/outcomes are met, it is possible that some will not be achieved before discharge. The goals/outcomes that have not been met need to be reviewed, and the reasons why documented. Some nursing diagnoses, such as Anxiety or Altered Nutrition, may require many months or years to be completely resolved. Since the hospitalization is only one point along the patient's health continuum, it is realistic that not all outcomes will be achieved or all nursing diagnoses resolved.

The discharge plans that began at the time of admission and were periodically updated are finalized and put into action. Verify that the patient/significant other have received written and verbal instructions regarding treatments, medications, and activities to be followed/referred to at home. Signs and symptoms indicating the need for continued contact with the healthcare providers are reviewed. When necessary, referral/contact phone numbers and other information about resources are given to the patient/significant other. You also determine whether contact has been made with appropriate providers for follow-up care as indicated (e.g., social worker, home health nurse, or equipment suppliers).

Concerns regarding unmet needs, the need for follow-up monitoring, and progress toward long-term goals after discharge were discussed in Chapter 4. Depending upon how your agency has decided to deal with these issues, you may choose to document your findings and patient instructions in a discharge summary, which also identifies additional activities for the patient and family to resolve unmet needs and achieve long-range outcomes/goals. A copy of this nursing discharge summary may then be given to the patient. Table 6–1 (see page 117) shows how patient teaching information can be organized and conveyed to the patient.

PLAN OF CARE: MICHELLE

Patient: Michelle   Age: 14 — 3/2/81   Sex: F   Admission: 6/11/95 5:30 PM   Dx: Compound Fx R tibia/fibula, closed head injury/mild concussion

Date	Patient Diagnostic Statement	Goal	Interventions	Outcomes	Status
6/11/95	Pain [acute], related to movement of bone fragments, soft tissue injury/edema and use of external fixator as evidenced by verbal reports, guarding, muscle tension narrowed focus, and tachycardia.	Pain-free or controlled by discharge.	1. Maintain limb rest R leg x 24 hr to 5 PM 6/12. 2. Elevate lower leg with folded blanket. 3. Apply ice to area as tolerated x 48 hr to 5 PM 6/13. 4. Place cradle over foot of bed. 5. Document reports and characteristics of pain. 6. Medicate with Demerol 75 mg and Phenergan 25 mg IM, q 4 hr prn or Vicodin 5 mg po q 4 hr prn. 7. Demonstrate/ encourage use of progressive relaxation techniques, deep-breathing exercises, visualization. 8. Provide alternate comfort measures, position change, backrub. 9. Encourage use of diversional activities.	Verbalizes relief of pain within 30 minutes of administration of medication. Identifies methods that provide relief by 9 AM, 6/12. Uses relaxation skills to reduce level of pain by 9 AM, 6/12.	
6/11/95	Infection, risk for, risk factors of broken skin, traumatized tissues, decreased hemoglobin levels, invasive	Free of infection	1. Monitor temp, V.S. q 4 hr. 2. Aseptic dressing change bid 9 AM, 9 PM, and prn.	Identifies and practices interventions to reduce risk of infection by 5 PM, 6/12.	

Date	Nursing Diagnosis	Interventions	Expected Outcomes
	procedures, environmental exposure.	3. Pin care per protocol bid 9 AM, 9 PM. 4. Routine IV site care daily. 5. Document condition of wound, IV, and pin sites q 4 hr. 6. Review ways patient can reduce risk of infection. 7. Administer cefoxitin 2 gm IV piggyback q 8 hrs (8 AM, 4 PM, 12 AM).	Identifies signs/symptoms requiring medical evaluation by 9 AM, 6/13. Achieves timely wound healing free of purulent drainage by discharge.
6/11/95	Physical mobility, impaired, related to musculoskeletal impairment and pain, and restrictive therapy (external fixator) as evidenced by reluctance to attempt movement and imposed restrictions of movement.	Ambulates safely with assistive device. 1. Monitor circulation/nerve function R leg q 1 hr x 24 hr, then q 4 hr and prn. 2. Support R leg fixator during movement. 3. Support feet with footboard. 4. Encourage use of side rails/overhead trapeze for position change. 5. Demonstrate/assist with ROM exercises to unaffected limbs 2 q hr. 6. Assist out of bed, non–weight-bearing R leg 6 PM, 6/12. 7. Instruct in/monitor use of crutches 6/13.	Participates in activities to maintain muscle strength by 9 AM, 6/12. Increases level of activity by 6 PM, 6/12. Demonstrates techniques/behaviors that enable resumption of activities by 6 PM, 6/13. Maintains position of function R leg, free of foot drop—ongoing.

PRACTICE ACTIVITY 6–1

EVALUATING PATIENT OUTCOMES

Read over the case study information below. It has been used to develop a plan of care for Michelle.

When Michelle was admitted to the hospital the evening of 6/11, a physiologic (Maslow's) or survival (Kalish) need of pain avoidance was identified (i.e., Pain [acute]). A higher-level problem of safety or stimulation was noted (i.e., Physical Mobility, impaired) as was a safety need of protection (i.e., Infection, risk for).

The following morning (6/12) during the 8 AM assessment, Michelle indicates she was successful in obtaining relief of pain after periodic injection of analgesics. Michelle also found that deep-breathing exercises and focusing her attention on the scenic picture at the foot of her bed helped to minimize the severity of recurrent muscle spasms in her right leg. In addition, frequent weight shifts using the overhead trapeze and range of motion exercises reduced general aches and joint stiffness.

The nurse noticed that most of Michelle's breakfast tray was untouched. Michelle reported she wan't very hungry but did want fruit juice and other fluids. After the morning bed bath, the dressings were changed and right leg wound was evaluated. Skin edges were pink and serous drainage was odorless. Pin sites were also cleaned and no signs of inflammation noted. At lunch, Michelle's intake was poor. She indicated she was having difficulty opening her mouth and chewing, and had an aching sensation located in right temple and ear.

During the afternoon assessment at 4:30 PM, Michelle's nurse verified that Michelle understood and was using infection control techniques of proper handwashing and avoidance of contact with wound and pin sites.

When Michelle was set up on the side of the bed before her dinner, she reported dizziness and sharp pain in her right leg, and she became pale and diaphoretic. She was returned to the supine position and a focused assessment was performed, revealing a blood pressure of 92/60. Within 20 minutes, Michelle's color had improved, the dizziness was gone, and the pain relieved with medication.

In reviewing the excerpts from Michelle's plan of care, complete the status column denoting whether the outcomes have been met (m), partially met (pm), or not met (nm) appropriately for the timeframes indicated.

PRACTICE ACTIVITY 6–2

MODIFICATION OF THE PLAN OF CARE

Based on your evaluation, how would you alter Michelle's plan of care from Practice Activity

6–1? _____

_____

_____

_____

Table 6–1 EXAMPLE OF PATIENT TEACHING INFORMATION FOR PATIENT GOING HOME ON ANTIDYSRHYTHMIC MEDICATION

Dear Patient:

This drug has been prescribed for you. This is what you should know about your drug to get the most from your therapy.

1. Antidysrhythmic medications are taken to regulate your heart rhythm.
2. Antidysrhythmic medications may have to be taken for the rest of your life.
3. Quinidine, procainamide hydrochloride (Pronestyl), propranolol (Inderal), and phenytoin (Dilantin) are taken with meals.
4. Do not take your antidysrhythmics concurrently with _____ [fill in appropriate drugs].
5. Always check with your doctor or pharmacist before taking other drugs because interactions may occur. Drugs known to cause interactions include over-the-counter products for nasal congestion, allergy, pain, or obesity. Drugs of abuse such as marijuana may raise the blood pressure and stimulate heart activity and thus increase abnormal heart rhythm.
6. If you forget to take your antidysrhythmic, do not take the forgotten dose. Do not try to catch up by taking 2 doses at the same time.
7. Do not stop taking your drug unless directed by your doctor.
8. If you have any side effects from your drug, call your doctor. Side effects from taking antidysrhythmics include low blood pressure, lightheadedness, gastrointestinal distress, changes in rate or rhythm of the heart, and often blurred vision. Keep a written record of specific effects that are noted and the time of day that they are noted, such as in the morning on awaking, with meals, or with activity. [List specific side effects for prescribed drug.]
9. Weigh yourself weekly. A gain of 1–2 lb a week may be a sign of increased water. Call your doctor if this occurs.
10. Check your feet and ankles for swelling. If this occurs, notify your doctor.
11. Limit your coffee, tea, or cola drinks, since caffeine may cause an increase in abnormal heart rhythm.
12. Store these drugs in a tight, light-resistant bottle to prevent deterioration.

Source: Reprinted from Mathewson-Kuhn, M. (1994). Pharmacotherapeutics: A Nursing Process Approach (3rd ed.). Philadelphia: F. A. Davis, with permission.

Even though the patient has been discharged, it is important for the patient and family to know what has been accomplished and how they can continue to enhance the patient's future health status. In addition, the discharge summary may be shared with the home care nurse/nurse practitioner and possibly sent to the primary/involved physician for inclusion in the office record to promote continuity of care with continued work toward goals and monitoring of progress/changing needs.

ENHANCING DELIVERY OF QUALITY CARE

Evaluation is an important step for determining the success of the plan of care because it involves a review of all the steps of the nursing process. Although patient care is evaluated on an individual basis, unit and/or general agency-based nursing audit committees focus attention on selected groups of patients, such as those receiving chemotherapy or those with longer than normal lengths of stay. Comparing overall outcomes and noting the effectiveness of specific interventions are the clinical components of evaluation that can become the bases of research for validating the nursing process. This external evaluation process is the key for refining standards of care and determining the protocols, policies, and procedures necessary for the provision of quality nursing care in a particular agency.

SUMMARY

The Evaluation step of the nursing process monitors and reports on the current status of the identified patient problems/needs and is based on the outcomes that were developed in the Planning step. The evaluation process includes the patient, significant others, and whoever else is involved in the care of the patient. This process is a positive one in which the patient's responses to the nursing interventions are evaluated to determine whether or not the desired outcomes were achieved. When the findings are analyzed and it is determined that the outcomes have been met, termination of services is begun and discharge planning is completed. However, if the outcomes have not been met (all or in part), reassessment is required to determine why this is the case. Consider factors, like new information, unexpected complications, or the choice of the wrong nursing diagnosis as possibilities when a desired patient outcome is not achieved. At this point, you would reinitiate the nursing process and modify the plan of care to include the newly identified nursing diagnoses, outcomes, and/or interventions. This modification, in turn, will be re-evaluated at an appropriate time.

The evaluation process can also be more broadly applied at an institutional level to measure the overall quality of care. It is increasingly used to set standards and to supply client information about many facets of the care provided by healthcare agencies. The Evaluation step needs to be viewed positively as an opportunity for growth, both for individuals and for the profession as a whole. It is essential for the effective delivery of patient care, and therefore a process to be valued rather than avoided and/or glossed over quickly.

Now, let us return to the sixth and last standard of the ANA Standard of Clinical Nursing Practice and review the measurement criteria necessary to achieve and ensure compliance. The knowledge and skill required to meet the

---

BOX 6–2 MEASUREMENT CRITERIA FOR ANA STANDARD VI

ANA Standard VI Evaluation: The nurse evaluates the client's progress toward attainment of outcomes.

Measurement Criteria

1. Evaluation is systematic and ongoing.
2. The client's responses to interventions are documented.
3. The effectiveness of interventions is evaluated in relation to outcomes.
4. Ongoing assessment data are used to revise diagnoses, outcomes, and the plan of care as needed.
5. Revisions in diagnoses, outcomes, and the plan of care are documented.
6. The client, significant others, and healthcare providers are involved in the evaluation process, when appropriate.

criteria listed in Box 6–2 were described in this chapter. The measurement criteria for this standard, combined with the previous standards, provide a valuable tool for evaluating your understanding and application of the nursing process.

Accurate documentation of the findings of the Evaluation step, is essential for ensuring the continuity of care described in the plan of care. This topic will be discussed in Chapter 7.

WORK PAGE: Chapter Six

1. What is the difference between assessment and evaluation? _____

_____

_____

2. What is the primary purpose of the evaluation process? _____

_____

3. The evaluation process provides what three opportunities for the patient and nurse:

a. _____

b. _____

c. _____

4. List the three methods in which patient outcomes may be evaluated, and give an example for each:

Method of Evaluation   **Example**

a. _____   _____

b. _____   _____

c. _____   _____

5. Because it is advisable to deal with only three to five nursing diagnoses at a time, how are needs

prioritized? _____

_____

6. When is consideration of discharge planning begun? _____

_____

7.

Vignette: Today is Donald's fifth hospital day. At the start of the shift, you have completed a focused assessment to evaluate progress/changes in status of the identified patient problems. Donald's initial nausea has resolved and his intake yesterday was approximately 3000 calories. During rounds you notice he has eaten all of the food on his breakfast tray. He fills out the next day's menu, neglecting to include any vegetables and selecting only one fruit.

Later, during group, Donald talks about his options for employment and says he knows an employment agency and a business where he can check about possible jobs. He also mentions a friend who he believes might be willing to help him. He says he is realizing that he is really OK, even though the loss of his job was a devastating event for him following so soon after his divorce. He acknowledges that his feelings of anxiety lead to an increase in his drinking. He further says he still has feelings of sadness and occasionally feels a sense of despair but believes he will feel better as he begins to get his life back together again. He seems tentative about accepting his need to be involved in AA, saying he doesn't know "where they meet, or anyone who attends the meetings."

a. **Evaluation:** Based on the above information, evaluate Donald's progress regarding his problems of Nutrition, altered, less than body requirements; Coping, Individual, ineffective; and Role Performance, altered, as outlined in the Plan of Care.

b. **Modification:** How would you change Donald's plan of care? _____

_____

_____

c. How might new concerns regarding the patient affect your discharge plans? _____

_____

BIBLIOGRAPHY

Carpenito, L.J. (1991). *Nursing Care Plans and Documentation.* Philadelphia: J.B. Lippincott.

Cox, H., et al. (1993). *Clinical Applications of Nursing Diagnosis: Adult Health, Child Health, Women's Health, Mental Health, and Home Health* (2nd ed.). Philadelphia: F.A. Davis.

Craft, M.J., & Denehy, J.A. (1990). *Nursing Interventions for Infants and Children.* Philadelphia: W.B. Saunders.

Doenges, M.E., & Moorhouse, M.F. (1993). *Nurse's Pocket Guide: Nursing Diagnoses with Interventions* (4th ed.). Philadelphia: F.A. Davis.

Doenges, M.E., Moorhouse, M.F., & Geissler, A.C. (1993). *Nursing Care Plans: Guidelines for Planning and Documenting Patient Care* (3rd ed.). Philadelphia: F.A. Davis.

Holloway, N.M. (1993). *Medical-Surgical Care Planning* (2nd ed.). Springhouse, PA: Springhouse.

Leuner, J.D., Manton, A.K., Kelliher, D.B., Sullivan, S.P., & Doherty, M. (1990). *Mastering the Nursing Process: A Case Study Approach.* Philadelphia: F.A. Davis.

Maas, M., Buckwalter, K.C., & Hardy, M. (1991). *Nursing Diagnosis and Interventions for the Elderly.* Menlo Park, CA: Addison-Wesley.

PLAN OF CARE: DONALD

Patient: Donald   Age: 46—2/4/48   Sex: M   Admission: 11/09/94 3:40 PM   Dx: Acute Alcoholism/Depression

Date	Patient Diagnostic Statement	Goal	Interventions	Outcomes	Status
11/09/94 Problem 4	Nutrition, altered, less than body requirements related to biologic, psychologic, and economic factors as evidenced by reported inadequate food intake, lack of interest in food, body weight 20 percent below ideal, and poor muscle tone.	*Short term:* Gains 1 to 2 lb/wk. *Long term:* Maintains weight between 160 and 170 pounds.	1. Weigh every other day (even) 7 AM. 2. Request evaluation by dietician 11/11. 3. Discuss individual dietary needs and ways to meet them. 4. Review daily dietary choices on patient's menu. 5. Calculate calorie count daily.	Verbalizes understanding of individual needs by 9 AM, 11/14. Intake meets minimum estimated requirements of 3000 cal/day by 9 AM, 11/14. Identifies ways of meeting nutritional needs within limits of financial resources by 9 AM, 11/15. Weight gain of 2 pounds by 8 AM, 11/16. *C. Walker, RN*	
11/12 Problem 5	Coping, Individual, ineffective, related to situational crisis of unemployment, recent divorce, personal vulnerability evidenced by reported inability to cope, use of alcohol, insomnia, and diminished problem-solving.	*Short term:* Dealing with current situation without reliance on alcohol. *Long term:* Expresses sense of self-worth. Maintains sobriety.	1. Assess level of anxiety and Donald's perception of situation. 2. Note verbal/nonverbal behaviors of anxiety. 3. Check on patient every 2 hr prn at irregular intervals. 4. Encourage verbalization, expression of feelings of denial/depression/anger. 5. Discuss normalcy of these feelings. 6. Identify current coping mechanisms.	Verbalizes awareness of sources of anxiety by 10 AM, 11/14. Demonstrates congruency between feelings/behavior by 10 AM, 11/15. Demonstrates initial problem-solving skills by 10 AM, 11/15. Identifies options and resources available for assistance by 10 AM, 11/16.	

(Continued)

PLAN OF CARE: DONALD (Continued)

Patient: Donald   Age: 46—2/4/48   Sex: M   Admission: 11/09/94 3:40 PM   Dx: Acute Alcoholism/Depression

Date	Patient Diagnostic Statement	Goal	Interventions	Outcomes	Status
			7. Note effectiveness/need for change.		
			8. Discuss/refer to resources: social worker, alcohol counselor, support group, AA.		
	Role Performance, altered, related to loss of job and recent divorce evidenced by change in perception of self as "ex"–husband, absent father; change in usual responsibilities, maladaptive coping (i.e., use of alcohol).	*Short term:* Accepting current situation. *Long term:* Assuming new roles in relation to ex-wife and relationship with children. Employed, meeting financial obligations.	1. Discuss perceptions and concerns about current situation (loss of job, change in relationship with ex-wife and children).	Verbalizes realistic perception and acceptance of self in changed roles related to losses by 10 AM, 11/14.	
			2. Acknowledge reality of grieving process related to losses (job/divorce). Assist patient to develop plan for employment.	Develops realistic plans with two strategies for job hunting by 10 AM, 11/14.	
			3. Makes own contacts regarding job possibilities and reports results.	Follows through on plan by 10 AM, 11/16.	
			4. Participate in family therapy sessions with ex-wife and children to develop new roles/relationships in changing situation.	*R. Smith, R.N.*	

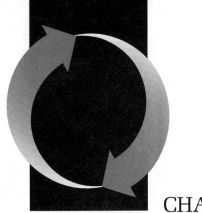

CHAPTER 7

Documenting the Nursing Process

■ **Role of Documentation**
■ **Progress Notes**
  Staff Communication
  Evaluation
  Relationship Monitoring
  Reimbursement
  Legal Documentation
  Accreditation
  Training and Supervision
■ **Techniques for Descriptive Note Writing**
  Judgmental Language
  Undefined Periods of Time
  Undefined Quantities
  Qualities
  Objective Basis for Judgments
  Descriptive Language
  Content of Note/Entry
  Format of Note/Entry
■ **Summary**

JCAHO Standard: Patient-Specific Data/Information

IM.7.1. A medical record is initiated and maintained for every individual assessed or treated. The medical record incorporates information from subsequent contacts between the patient and the organization.

IM.7.2. The medical record contains sufficient information to identify the patient, support the diagnosis, justify the treatment, document the course and results accurately, and facilitate continuity of care among healthcare providers.

ROLE OF DOCUMENTATION

Remember, for legal purposes, if an event/activity is not documented, it did not occur or was not done.

Documentation is not only a requirement for accreditation but is also a legal requirement in any healthcare setting. From a nursing focus, documentation provides a record of the use of the nursing process for the delivery of individualized patient care. The initial *assessment* is recorded in the patient history or data base.

The *identification* of patient problems/needs, and the *planning* of patient care are recorded in the plan of care. The *implementation* of the plan is recorded in the progress notes and/or flow sheets. Finally, the *evaluation* of care may be documented in the progress notes and/or plan of care.

The goals of the documentation system are to:

- Facilitate the delivery of quality patient care.
- Ensure documentation of progress with regard to patient-focused outcomes.
- Facilitate interdisciplinary consistency and the communication of treatment goals and progress.

PROGRESS NOTES

The plan of care that has been developed for a particular patient serves as a framework or outline for the charting of administered care. As noted, this information may be recorded on flow sheets and/or progress notes. Progress notes are an integral component of the overall medical record and should include all significant events that occur during the patient's hospitalization/treatment program. The notes should be written in a clear and objective fashion and in a manner that reflects progress towards desired measurable outcomes with the use of planned staff interventions. Progress notes have seven major functions as noted in Box 7–1.

BOX 7–1   SEVEN FUNCTIONS OF PROGRESS NOTES

Progress notes serve multiple functions, and any given note may be written to address one function more than the others. Thus it is important to recognize the seven major functions of progress notes:

1. Staff documentation
2. Evaluation
3. Relationship monitoring
4. Reimbursement
5. Legal documentation
6. Accreditation
7. Training and supervision

Staff Communication

Clearly, staff arriving on the next and subsequent shifts need to know what has been occurring with the patient during the current shift, in order to make appropriate judgments regarding patient management. Colleague-to-colleague communication is the most obvious function of the progress note, yet it is only a piece of the communication picture. Nursing staff are in the unique position of being in contact with the patient for extended periods of time and in a variety of situations. As a nurse, your observations of your patient's behavior and response to therapy provide invaluable information to the physician or other providers who may only see the patient for a few minutes each day. Whether or not the patient's current desired measurable outcomes and interventions are discontinued or revised, or new ones developed, depend on the information gathered.

Evaluation

Periodic review of the patient's progress and the effectiveness of the treatment plan is completed by the nurse and/or the treatment team. An evaluation of the patient's progress may be documented on the plan of care and/or in the progress notes.

For the purpose of review (for example, nursing audit committees and state, federal, and private agencies such as the Board of Health, Medicare, Joint Committee on the Accreditation of Healthcare Organizations [JCAHO]), the medical record should be written to facilitate an assessment of the care given the patient. Progress notes need to be written to reflect the patient's progress toward measurable outcomes and the interventions used. Someone not associated with the healthcare facility should be able to read the notes, determine if the plan of care is being implemented, and whether progress is being made toward the measurable outcomes. The medical record should serve as a method of tracking the patient's response to treatment and, consequently, as a means for evaluating the quality of care provided.

Relationship Monitoring

The therapeutic relationship existing between staff and patient is an important aspect of treatment in any setting. The NURSE-PATIENT RELATIONSHIP is the tool used by the nurse to help the patient make the most of his or her own abilities. In the psychiatric setting, many of the patient's pathologies are manifested in these relationships, and indications of progress are first identified through the patient's ability to relate more positively and openly with staff as well as peers and family. Therefore, monitoring the patient's relationships is essential, and notes detailing observations of these relationships (how the patient interacts in group situations, competitive situations, in one-to-one situations, etc.) have important clinical implications.

NURSE/PATIENT RELATIONSHIP—a therapeutic relationship built on a series of interactions, developing over time, and meeting the needs of the patient.

Reimbursement

Third-party reimbursers are insistent that the *why, when, where, how, what,* and *who* of services be clearly documented. An absence of such documentation may result in termination of funding for individual patients and, therefore, termination of treatment. The medical record is a primary source for maintaining the revenues as well as information about the patient's treatment, providing proof of services. Therefore, progress notes must document any significant observations about what is happening to the patient during illness, treatment, and recovery. Data about medications, equipment used, and any other pertinent information also needs to be recorded.

Legal Documentation

Nurses have a legal and moral duty to do no harm to patients. Harm can result from a nurse's action *or* inaction. Careful attention to all the steps of the nursing process reduce the possibility that harm will result from errors of omission (failing to take appropriate action as a result of missing an actual nursing diagnosis) or errors of commission (taking inappropriate action because of incorrect or overdiagnosing).

In our litigious society, with the threat of malpractice lawsuits, all aspects of the medical record (including the information contained in daily progress notes) may be important for legal documentation. Both the implementation of interventions and progress toward the measurable outcomes should be documented in the progress notes of the patient's medical record. Progress notes and flow sheets need to document that appropriate actions have been carried out and precautions taken as required to implement the treatment plan. These notations need to be specific about date and time and be signed by the person making the entry. In addition, the time an entry is written needs to be noted, along with the time the activity *actually* occurred when charting is delayed. Errors in the document must be crossed out with one line so that it is still legible, identified by the author as an "error," and then initialed. White-outs or cross-outs that make the information unreadable are not acceptable, as they could be construed to mean that the individual or facility is trying to alter the facts.

Accreditation

One of the most essential requirements for healthcare facilities (as determined by JCAHO and/or other accreditation and licensing agencies) is to maintain a medical record. JCAHO standards state that the medical record be documented accurately and in a timely manner. Therefore, the importance of completing notes on schedule and in a manner that facilitates retrieval of data should be emphasized. In addition, the JCAHO standards specify that "Nursing care data related to patient assessments, nursing diagnoses and/or patient needs, nursing interventions, and patient outcomes are permanently integrated into the medical record."

Training and Supervision

An often underestimated aspect of note writing is their value for training and supervision purposes. An experienced nurse's description of how a complicated situation was handled, a supervisor's analysis of the problems presented by a new admission, and a description of patterns noted in another patient's response to care are all examples of notes that provide models for the remainder of the staff. Supervisors also gain an insight into the employee's abilities through reading progress notes and may be able to isolate areas in which additional supervision or training/education would be beneficial.

Finally, regardless of the setting, the patient's relationship with significant other(s) can have an impact on general well-being, progress toward recovery, independence in self-care, and (ultimately) a successful transition to the home setting. Thus, observation and monitoring of these interactions are important components of nursing care. At this point, complete Practice Activity 7–1 before proceeding to the next section.

TECHNIQUES FOR DESCRIPTIVE NOTE WRITING

Potential readership for notes written in the medical record might include coworkers, clinical specialist nurses, nurse practitioners, physicians, therapists, psychiatrists, psychologists, social workers, nurse reviewers, lawyers, judges, utilization reviewers, insurance personnel, surveyors, agency representatives, parents or guardians, as well as the patient. Because of the number of possible readers, the need for clarity and accuracy in the progress notes is a priority.

From the notes, the reader should be able to form a clear picture of what occurred with the patient. The best way to ensure the clarity of progress notes is through the use of descriptive (or observational) statements. The following guideline for writing observation-based notes compares and contrasts judgmental and descriptive language.

Judgmental Language

We are all aware of the possibilities for miscommunication that exist in ordinary conversations. The dangers of miscommunication may be even greater when information is written, and the opportunities for clarification present in face-to-face communication are absent. We are accustomed to speaking and writing in a judgmental (and therefore ambiguous) manner without even being aware of it. Examples are noted in Box 7–2 (see page 132). Types of judgmental statements include phrases that:

- Make reference to undefined periods of time
- Refer to undefined quantities
- Refer to qualities
- Fail to specify any objective basis for the judgment made

Undefined Periods of Time

Statements that refer to undefined periods of time may contain words or phrases such as the following:

often	almost always	most of the time
rarely	frequently	now and then
seldom	occasionally	every so often

PRACTICE ACTIVITY 7-1

ELEMENTS OF PROGRESS NOTES

Give a brief explanation of how progress notes provide for the following elements of the nurse/patient relationship.

1. Staff communication: _____

_____

_____

2. Evaluation: _____

_____

_____

3. Relationship monitoring: _____

_____

_____

4. Reimbursement: _____

_____

_____

5. Legal documentation: _____

_____

_____

6. Accreditation: _____

_____

_____

7. Training/Supervision: _____

_____

_____

_____

Use of these and similar phrases without clarification may leave the statement unclear and judgmental. How often, for example, is "every so often"? Is it every 5 minutes, once an hour, or three times per shift? This is not to say that the staff member must time each and every interaction or occurrence. Rather, be aware of the *potential* for confusion in these words. Ask yourself: Do I need to be more specific about the time of the event mentioned in this note? If you are documenting for potential legal purposes (an injury, for example), specificity will be essential; however, for routine communication purposes, this may not be the case. For example, if you note "The patient was quiet for most of the shift today," the exact number of minutes during which she was quiet or not quiet is not necessary for reasonably accurate communication to occur.

Undefined Quantities

Statements that refer to undefined quantities may use such words or phrases as the following:

some	enough	a greal deal	too much
a lot	many	very little	large amount

As with the previous statements, each of these terms is open to interpretation. "A lot" of complaints to one person, for example, might mean 5; to another it might mean 20. Or, "a moderate amount of bloody drainage" could be 200 mL or only 50 mL of fluid. It is generally advisable to avoid undefined quantities.

Qualities

All descriptive adjectives applied to patients have the potential to fall under this category, since they may involve making subjective definitions beforehand. Of most concern, however, are words that could be called "semitechnical" in nature:

passive	irritating	incompetent
nervous	manipulative	overprotective
demanding	alcoholic	disturbed

Because these kinds of words have connotations in the health field beyond the scope of their ordinary definitions, more common adjectives may pose less of a problem because there is less potential for misunderstanding. However, observed behaviors may call for conclusions that are influenced by your own biases and cultural background. It is best to verify the connotations of the following terms with others and particularly with the patient before using them:

friendly	unhappy	enthusiastic	proud
attentive	excited	bored	observant
aloof	apathetic	cheerful	happy

Finally, there are slang words (used informally), which because they are used mostly by small subcultural groups, are unclear and should not be contained in a professionally written note in any case. For example:

hyped-up	spaced-out	bummed	crazy
loose	pushy	cool	tanked-up

BOX 7-2   EXAMPLES OF JUDGMENTAL LANGUAGE

Consider the following statements:

"He asks for pain medication *too often*."
"He is *uncooperative* today."
"She did a *good job* on her incentive spirometer today."
"He is a *manipulative* patient."
"The new patient is really *difficult*."
"He has a *poor* outlook."
"She had a *bad attitude* about doing her physical therapy this morning."

The highlighted words in each of the above statements represent judgments (or conclusions), not facts. Without any elaboration or basis for comparison, each of the statements is a statement of opinion, open to varying interpretations. Contrast these with the statements in Box 7-3.

Objective Basis for Judgments

Some statements are clearly a judgment on the part of the observer and are offered without any objective basis. Such statements may cause the reader to ask "How do you *know* this patient . . ."

- is improving?
- has a good attitude?
- enjoys reading?
- hates his roommate?

Recording your observations and providing an objective basis for your judgment (as in Box 7-3) will reduce the possibility of miscommunication or misinterpretation, and the reader will not have to look elsewhere for clarification.

BOX 7-3   PROVIDING AN OBJECTIVE BASIS FOR YOUR JUDGMENTS

Consider the following statements. Although the highlighted words represent a judgment or conclusion, objective facts or behavioral observations are provided to support or substantiate the judgment.

Michelle *is improving*; she walked the length of the hall using her crutches unassisted.
Robert *has a good attitude*, expressing optimism that he will be able to prevent a recurrence of pneumonia.
Sally *enjoys reading*, spending 1 to 2 hours a day in this activity.
Donald *expresses anger* toward his roommates' smoking, loud conversations with visitors, and commandeering of the TV. (Note: Making the inference that Donald *hates his roommate* from his expression of anger results in an unclear or unsupported judgment.)

Descriptive Language

As noted previously, descriptive language contains observations only and avoids statements that are evaluative or judgmental unless observational evidence can be presented to back up the judgment. You will remember that being able to actually observe the patient doing something was the criterion of a well-written outcome. The situation is similar for observation-based progress notes; properly written objective statements refer to specific observable or measurable events. Descriptive statements:

- *Contain measurable periods of time*

    For example:

ten times in 1 hour	every half hour	15 minutes
48 hours	four times a day	once

- *Contain measurable quantities*

    For example:

twenty percent of the diet	all of the patients
six out of eight	completely saturated
none	5 mL

- *Provide a basis or rationale for qualities named in the note*

    For example:

    Sally's lochia flow is moderate to heavy, saturating one peri-pad in approximately 1 hour on two separate occasions.

    Donald's intake at lunch was poor, consisting of 1/2 cup of soup, 2 bites of sandwich, and 1/2 glass of milk.

You may have gotten the impression in the preceding section that you can never use adjectives in your notes. This is far from the case. In fact, you should give your impressions of the patient.

Statements in which you note that the patient "seemed" or "appeared" to be exhibiting a certain physical/emotional state are inferential statements. These are a subset of descriptive statements in which you infer the patient's state based on your observations of the patient's behavior and interactions, your knowledge of the patient's patterns, and the connections you make between behavior/affect and what has been happening during the illness. Such statements are often of great value.

However, you do not allow your subjective impressions to stand alone, particularly if your observation involves some of the more "semitechnical" qualities noted earlier. You also need to provide some reasons why you believed the patient was "improving," "demanding," "manipulative," or whatever.

For example:

Robert was upset by his daughter's objections to his advance directive choices, cutting off the discussion and instructing her to "mind her own business."

Donald is passive, responding to the nurse's questions regarding scheduling of his care by replying "whatever you want to do."

Sally appears distressed, expressing concern about how she will manage two newborns when she already has two children at home, needs to return to work, and has no energy to do anything.

Michelle's mother is demanding, asking frequently for immediate nursing attention for minor needs.

When comparisons or judgments are made, a descriptive statement should state the source or basis of judgment.

For example:

According to the patient's laboratory reports . . .
Psychologic testing showed that . . .
The other patient stated that . . .
Judging by the fact that . . .

Also note that whenever the source of a judgment is specified, the statement becomes a behavioral report. Because such a report can be observed, this type of statement is an observation and is therefore descriptive. Consider the differences between the following two statements.

For example:

The patient is stronger today.
The physical therapist reports, "Michelle is stronger today."

BOX 7–4 COMPARISON OF JUDGMENTAL AND BEHAVIORAL NOTES

The important thing to know about judgmental statements is that they can be translated into more precise terms. For example:

Judgmental: The patient did pretty well today.
Behavioral: The patient followed directions for drawing up and administering his insulin without any mistakes.
Judgmental: The meeting with the physical therapist did not go very well.
Behavioral: The patient stated she "could not do the exercises which were to be started today."
Judgmental: The patient had a bad attitude all day.
Behavioral: The patient argued with staff five times during the shift.
Judgmental: The patient became aggressive.
Behavioral: The patient clenched his fists and yelled at the nurse, "I'd like to hit you." He then hit the wall twice with his fist.
Judgmental: The patient would not follow directions.
Behavioral: The patient drank a glass of water 30 minutes before his scheduled surgery in spite of reminders to remain NPO.
Judgmental: The patient ate poorly.
Behavioral: Patient ate one third of her lunch (all of the broccoli and corn, no meat, potatoes, or bread) and drank 50 mL of apple juice.

As you can see from the above examples, it often takes a bit more thought to write a note which is objectively descriptive. However, the benefits in clarity of communication make the effort essential for the many purposes of progress notes.

The first statement is clearly judgmental because of the undefined phrase "stronger today." The second, however, is an observable event. Obviously (although the physical therapist may be wrong) it is an objective fact that the physical therapist said that the patient is stronger today. It may help to think of such statements as quotations. What the physical therapist said does not influence our ability to observe him or her saying it, and then objectively reporting that observation. However, physical therapy notes should reflect measurable descriptions of the patient situation.

Finally, you can chart observations in a nonjudgmental manner. "Michelle displayed increased endurance, walked the length of hall without assistance, appeared more confident with crutch use." In Box 7−4, additional examples further illustrate how judgmental statements may be interpreted and restated more objectively. To further assist you in your understanding of documenting descriptive progress notes, take a moment to complete Practice Activity 7−2.

Content of Note/Entry

The term *progress note* indicates that the patient's progress is to be documented along with the implementation of the treatment plan. Contents should be as specific and accurate as possible.

For communication purposes, it is important to record in the progress notes any information that is of importance to oncoming shifts as well as observations you have made which may be significant for other healthcare providers. Box 7−5 (see page 137) profiles what information should be included. Remember, you are actually charting for the future. You know what is happening today. However, the reader of tomorrow, next week, or next year must rely on your written words in order to share your understanding of the patient's situation at a given moment.

For example, when applying restraints (which constitutes a "major event with both therapeutic and legal ramifications"), you need to document the exact time the procedure was initiated, whether any injuries resulted, and so forth. It is also necessary to document what led up to the situation, how staff and other participants reacted, what less restrictive measures were tried, and any significant observations regarding the incident. An example of how to document a therapeutic event is presented in Box 7−6 (see page 137).

Other areas of concern that enhance accurate communication are the use of correct grammar and spelling, legible writing, and the use of nonerasable ink. To promote clarity, avoid repeating data when possible. Since this is "the patient's record," it is not necessary to use the term "the patient"; however, periodically using the patient's name can help to identify the proper chart and prevent problems of charting on the wrong record, especially when you chart on several patient's records at a time. Use abbreviations with caution or avoid them in most instances. Although some institutions provide a list of approved abbreviations that identifies the correct meaning (such as those included in Appendix G), abbreviations can be misleading or easily misinterpreted, resulting in misunderstandings and errors with serious consequences. For example, a patient reading his record might not realize that "SOB" stands for short of breath.

Last, but not least, remember to be brief. Entries need to be concise, short,

PRACTICE ACTIVITY 7–2

WRITING NONJUDGMENTAL STATEMENTS

Circle either the **J** *or* **O/B** *for each of the following statements to identify either judgmental* (**J**) *or observational/behavioral* (**O/B**) *documented statements. If the statement is judgmental rewrite to reflect observational/behavioral language.*

1. Mrs. Jewel has a poor body image since undergoing a mastectomy.   J   O/B   _____

_____

2. Mr. Dunn needs to be evaluated regarding his competence to manage his household affairs

due to his left-sided weakness since his stroke.   J   O/B   _____

_____

3. Miss Janus does a good job of breast self-examination.   J   O/B   _____

_____

4. Mary Bird does not eat enough for her current level of activity.   J   O/B   _____

_____

5. Mr. Lambert stops taking his medication; then when he has a seizure, he presents at the doc-

tor's office for treatment.   J   O/B   _____

_____

6. It has been a long time since Mr. Babbitt has had his medications evaluated.   J   O/B

_____

_____

succinct sentences or phrases that provide enough information to communicate your observations, thoughts, and plans. The entry needs to be consistent in style and format to avoid confusion and comply with agency policies. Avoid repetition/redundancy. Do not rewrite what is already recorded on flow sheets, but do use the progress note to expand on the flow sheet as appropriate and to note the patient's response. For example: when documenting your repeat assessment of a wound, you may chart "no change" (if that is the case) if your baseline or previous observations are recorded.

BOX 7–5   CONTENT OF SUCCESSFUL PROGRESS NOTES

Examples of the kind of information important to record in the progress notes include:

- *Unsettled or unclear problems or "issues"* that need to be dealt with, including attempts to contact other healthcare providers
- *Noteworthy incidents or interviews* involving the patient that would benefit from a more detailed recording
- *Other pertinent data* such as notes on phone calls, home visits, and family interactions
- *Additional critical incident data* such as seemingly significant or revealing statements made by the patient, an insight you have into a patient's patterns of behavior, patient injuries, the use of any special treatment procedure, or other major events such as episodes of pain, respiratory distress, panic attacks, medication reactions, suicidal comments
- *Administered cure activities or observations* if not recorded elsewhere on flow sheets (physician visits, completion of ordered tests, nonroutine medications, etc.)

BOX 7–6   DOCUMENTING A THERAPEUTIC EVENT

Twenty-four hours after Donald was admitted to the unit with a diagnosis of acute alcoholism, he became disoriented to time, place, and person; was extremely agitated; and was "picking in the air" saying he was trying to "catch the bugs." He was given medication and placed in restraints in a seclusion room with the door open. This was charted as follows:

4:00 PM: Became agitated without notice. Medicated with Valium, reoriented to place/events in quiet tones as staff paced with him, and reinforced that he would be kept safe. Agitation escalated, unable to remain in one place for longer than 60 seconds, expressed fear of the "things" he was seeing. Agreed to use of restraints to help keep him safe until he could regain control and/or medication becomes effective.

4:15 PM: Procedure explained as Donald was put in seclusion room C and placed in 4-point wrist/ankle restraints without incident or injury. Informed that door would remain open and a staff member would check on him every 10 minutes or more frequently as needed. Vital signs: B/P 150/90, P 120. Respirations 32.

4:20 PM: Dr. Carter notified of current status.

> **BOX 7–7 COMPONENTS OF THE SOAP/SOAPIER CHARTING FORMAT**
>
> The **SOAP** format is generally used for the initial assessment of the patient. Once the plan of care is implemented and the evaluation process begun, the **SOAPIER** format becomes more appropriate.
>
> **S**ubjective: statements from patient/others
> **O**bjective: measurable or observable data
> **A**nalysis: interpretations/conclusions based on the subjective and/or objective data
> **P**lan: what is to be done about the identified problem(s)
> **I**mplementation: how plan is carried out
> **E**valuation: patient's response to the interventions
> **R**evision: how the plan of care will be changed

Format of Note/Entry

POMR OR PORS—Problem Oriented Medical Record—a method of recording data about the health status of the patient by focusing on the patient's problems.

There are several charting formats that have been used for documentation. These include: block notes, with a single entry covering an entire shift (e.g., 7–3 PM); narrative timed notes (e.g., 8:30 AM, Ate all of breakfast); and the problem-oriented medical record system (POMR or PORS) using the SOAP/SOAPIER approach (Box 7–7), to name a few. The last format can provide thorough documentation, but it was designed by physicians for episodic care and requires that the entries be tied to a patient problem identified from a problem list.

SOAP/SOAPIER—format for documentation—subjective, objective, analysis, plan; implementation, evaluation, revision.

A new system format created by nurses for documentation of frequent/repetitive care is FOCUS Charting™. It was designed to encourage looking at the patient from a positive rather than a negative (or problem-oriented) perspective by using precise documentation to record the nursing process. Recording of assessment, interventions, and evaluation information in a DAR (Data, Action, and Response) format (Box 7–8) facilitates tracking and following what is happening to the patient at any given moment. Charting focuses on patient and nursing concerns. The focal point is patient status and the associated nursing care. The "Focus" is always stated to reflect the patient's con-

DAR—format for documentation—data, action, response.

> **BOX 7–8 COMPONENTS OF THE FOCUS CHARTING™ FORMAT**
>
> **Focus:** Nursing diagnosis. patient problem/concern, sign/symptom, event
>
>   **D**ata: Subjective/objective information describing and/or supporting the focus
>
>   **A**ction: Immediate/future nursing actions based on assessment and consistent with/complimentary to the goals and nursing action recorded in the patient plan of care
>
>   **R**esponse: Describes the effects of interventions and whether or not the goal/outcome was met

cern/need rather than a nursing task or medical diagnosis. Box 7−9 highlights some of the distinguishing features of a Focus.

Whatever documentation system you use, an organized format is a method of identifying, working through, and solving the patient's problems. SOAP and DAR help to organize your thinking and provide structure, which can promote creative problem solving. Structured communication facilitates consistency between various services and healthcare providers. Compare the charts in Tables 7−1 (see page 141) and 7−2 (see page 142) for a NIDDM patient (non−insulin dependent diabetes mellitus), with an ulceration of the left foot.

A copy of the back page of the interactive plan of care worksheet is included in Figure 7−1 (see page 143). It is an example of one method of documenting by focusing on certain aspects of the nursing process. The DOCU-MENTATION section of the interactive plan of care worksheet is divided into three possible areas where documentation is appropriate and may be required in certain agencies. The first section is reassessment data. In this area you will review the patient's initial assessment data to note any changes. Also, data derived from MONITORING focused nursing interventions ("monitor vital signs every shift" or "monitor serum potassium level every eight hours") are documented in this section. The second documentation area directs attention to the nursing interventions implemented to assist patients in attaining their stated desired outcome. Examples may include "Assisted patient with ambulation bid" or "Instructed in proper use of a walker." Finally, the third section is the patient's response to your interventions: How well did the patient tolerate his assisted ambulation? Or, did the patient use the walker in the correct manner as demonstrated?

SUMMARY

Documentation of patient care communicates and reflects the individualization of care you provide. Documentation promotes continuity of patient care among the varied healthcare providers and serves as a basis for the evaluation of the care provided. Finally, the documentation process continually reinforces your accountability and responsibility to implement and evaluate the nursing process. As your documentation skills improve, you will save time by consistently using a documentation system that focuses on specific issues. Accurate documentation can also help in meeting legal and accreditation requirements.

The last chapter in this text includes a patient case study to help you bring all the steps of the nursing process together. The case study includes information about a new patient, Mr. R. Simmons. His completed nursing data base and the physician's admitting orders are provided to assist you in identifying possible nursing diagnoses, developing appropriate desired outcomes for Mr. Simmons, and selecting nursing interventions that will assist him in attaining the desired outcomes.

The final chapter also presents an evaluation checklist that was developed to include the important aspects of all of the American Nurses' Association ANA's standards of clinical nursing practice detailed throughout this text. This comprehensive evaluation checklist serves as a helpful tool for your self-evaluation and ensures that your assigned written care planning efforts are correctly accomplished.

BOX 7-9 WHAT IS A FOCUS?

The nurse often speaks of "a focus" for her assessment, diagnosis, and planning of care.

- A patient problem/concern or nursing diagnosis,

  For example:

  Airway   Nutrition   Fluid excess
  Knowledge deficit: wound care

  The "stem" or diagnostic label is taken from the plan of care. You do not need to use time and space to repeat the entire diagnostic statement.

- Signs/symptoms of potential importance.

  For example:

  fever   confusion
  hypotension   nausea
  dysrhythmia   edema

  These require monitoring or limited intervention, but if the signs and symptoms persist, a patient problem will be identified and added to the plan of care.

  For example:

  continued nausea can affect fluid volume; dysrhythmias and hypotension may develop into a cardiac output concern.

- Significant event or change in status.

  For example:

  admission/transfer   seizure activity
  fall out of bed   respiratory arrest

- A single incident may evolve into a patient problem for inclusion in the plan of care.

  For example:

  a fall raises concerns about Injury, risk for, or possibly, Thought Processes, altered, if patient is disoriented; or a respiratory arrest may be related to Airway Clearance, ineffective, or Breathing Pattern, ineffective.

- Specific standards of care/hospital policy

  For example:

  admission/discharge   preoperative visit
     summary   discharge planning
  routine shift assessment

Table 7–1 SAMPLE SOAP/IER CHARTING FORMAT FOR RICHARD

DATE	TIME	NUMBER/PROBLEM*	SOAP FORMAT†
6/30/94	1400	1 (Skin Integrity)	**S:** "That hurts" (when tissue surrounding wound palpated). **O:** Scant amount serous drainage on dressing. Wound borders pink. No odor present. **A:** Wound shows early signs of healing, free of infection. **P:** Continue skin care per plan of care.

In order to document more of the nursing process, some institutions have added the following: Implementation, Evaluation, and Revision (if plan was altered)

			I: Betadine soaks as ordered. Applied sterile dressing with paper tape. **E:** Wound clean, no drainage present. Signed: *E. Moore R.N*
6/28/94	2100	2 (Pain)	**S:** "Dull, throbbing pain (in left foot)," says there is no radiation to other areas. **O:** Muscles tense. Moving about bed, appears uncomfortable. **A:** Persistent pain. **P:** Foot cradle placed on bed. Darvon 65 mg given po. Signed: *M. Siskin R.N*
	2130		**E:** Reports pain relieved. Appears relaxed. Signed: *B. Marsh R.N*
6/30/94	1100	3 (Knowledge deficit, diabetic teaching)	**S:** Listed questions/concerns of self and wife. (Copy attached to teaching plan.) **O:** None **A:** Richard and wife need review of information and practice for insulin administration. **P:** Attend group teaching session with wife and meet with dietitian. Read <u>Understanding Your Diabetes.</u> **I:** He demonstrated insulin administration technique for wife to observe. Procedure handout sheet for future reference provided to couple. Scheduled meeting for them with dietitian at 1300 today to discuss remaining questions. **E:** Richard more confident in demonstration, performed activity without hesitation, correctly and without hand tremors. Richard explained steps of procedure and reasons for actions to wife. Couple identified resources to contact if questions/problems arise. Signed: *B. Briner, R.N*

* As noted on Plan of Care.
† S = Subjective: statements from patient/others.
  O = Objective: measurable or observable data.
  A = Analysis: interpretations/conclusions based on the subjective and/or objective data.
  P = Plan: what is to be done about the identified problem(s).
  I = Implementation: how plan is carried out.
  E = Evaluation: patient's response to the interventions.
  R = Revision: how the plan of care will be changed.

Table 7–2   SAMPLE OF DAR FOR RICHARD

DATE	TIME	FOCUS	DAR FORMAT*
6/30/94	1400	Skin integrity L foot	**D:** Scant amount serous drainage on dressing, wound borders pink, no odor present, denies discomfort except with direct palpation of surrounding tissue **A:** Betadine soak as ordered. Sterile dressing applied with paper tape **R:** Wound clean—no drainage present. Signed: *E. Moore RN*
6/28/94	2100	Pain L foot	**D:** "Reports dull/throbbing ache L foot—no radiation. Muscles tense, restless in bed. **A:** Foot cradle placed on bed. Darvon 65 mg given po. Signed: *M. Siskin RN*
	2200	Pain L foot	**R:** Reports pain relieved. Appears relaxed. Signed: *B. Marsh RN*
6/30/94	1100	Knowledge deficit, Diabetic teaching	**D:** Attended group teaching session with wife. Both have read *Understanding Your Diabetes*. **A:** Reviewed list of questions/concerns from Richard and wife. (Copy attached to teaching plan.) Richard demonstrated insulin administration technique for wife to observe. Procedure handout sheet for future reference provided to couple. Scheduled meeting for them with dietitian at 1300 today to discuss remaining questions. **R:** Richard more confident in demonstration, performed activity without hesitation, correctly and without hand tremors. He explained steps of procedure and reasons for actions to wife. Couple identified resources to contact if questions/problems arise. Signed: *B. Briner, RN*

The following is an example of documentation of a patient need/concern that currently does not require identification as a patient problem (nursing diagnosis) or inclusion in the plan of care and therefore not easily documented in the SOAP format:

6/29/94	2020	Gastric distress	**D:** Awakened, from light sleep by "indigestion/burning sensation." Places hand over epigastric area. Skin warm/dry, color pink, vital signs unchanged. **A:** Given Mylanta 30 mL po. Head of bed elevated approximately 15 degrees. **R:** Reports pain relieved. Appears relaxed, resting quietly. Signed: *E. Moore, RN*

* D = Data: subjective/objective information describing and/or supporting the focus.
  A = Action: immediate or future nursing actions that address the focus, any changes required for the plan of care.
  R = Response: description of patient responses to care provided and whether goals/outcomes are met.
Source: FOCUS Charting™, Susan Lampe, RN, MS, Creative Nursing Management, Inc., 614 East Grant Street, Minneapolis, MN 55404.

Desired Outcome and Patient Criteria: The Patient will:

TIME OUT! The desired outcome must meet criteria to be accurate. The outcome must be specific, realistic, measurable, and include a time frame for completion. Does the action verb describe the patient's behavior to be evaluated? Can the outcome be used in the evaluation step of the nursing process to measure the patient's response to the nursing interventions listed below?

Interventions	Rationale for Selected Intervention and References

P L A N N I N G

TIME OUT! Do your interventions assist in achieving the desired outcome? Do your interventions address further monitoring of the patient's response to your interventions and to the achievement of the desired outcome? Are qualifiers: **when, how, amount, time,** and **frequency** used? Is the focus of the action's verb on the nurse's actions and not on the patient? Do your rationales provide sufficient reason and directions?

What was your patient's response to the interventions?

Was the desired outcome achieved? ☐ Yes ☐ No   If no, what revisions to either the desired outcome or interventions would you make?

E V A L U A T I O N

Documentation Focus: Now that you have completed the evaluation, the next step is to document your care and the patient's response. Use the areas below to enter your progress note information.

Reassessment Data:

Interventions Implemented:

Patient's Response:

D O C U M E N T A T I O N

INSTRUCTOR'S COMMENTS:

Figure 7–1. Reverse side of the interactive care plan worksheet previously introduced, providing for documentation of the nursing process.

WORK PAGE: Chapter Seven

1. You are writing a paper regarding documentation. Identify three goals of the documentation process you will include:

a. _____

b. _____

c. _____

2. Steps of the nursing process are documented on which form:

Steps	**Form**
_____ Assessment	a. Plan of care
_____ Problem identification	b. Progress notes
_____ Planning	c. Patient data base
_____ Implementation	d. Flow sheets
_____ Evaluation	

3. List five functions of progress notes:

a. _____

b. _____

c. _____

d. _____

e. _____

4. Complete the following statements describing the JCAHO's standards for documentation.

a. A medical record is _____ and _____ for every individual assessed or

treated. The medical record incorporates information from subsequent contacts between the

_____ and _____ .

b. The medical record contains _____ _____ to _____ the pa-

tient, support the _____ , justify the _____ , document the course and

results accurately, and facilitate _____ of care among healthcare providers.

5. When documenting for reimbursement, five factors need to be included. These are: _____

_____

_____

6. Two ways in which the plan of care can be used for supervision are: _____

_____

7. The best way to ensure clarity of the progress notes is: _____

_____

8. Rewrite the following judgmental statements to make them nonjudgmental:

a. He is uncooperative today. _____

_____

b. He is a manipulative patient. _____

_____

c. She had a bad attitude about taking her medication this morning. _____

_____

d. The new patient is really difficult. _____

_____

9. List three types of judgmental statements:

a. _____

b. _____

c. _____

10. Name three types of data which are important to record in the progress notes:

a. _____

b. _____

c. _____

11. List five additional factors that can enhance accurate communication:

a. _____

b. _____

c. _____

d. _____

e. _____

12. What actions can be taken to correct an error in charting? _____

_____

13. Name three charting formats:

   a. _____   b. _____   c. _____

14. Read the following Vignette and record the patient data using the SOAP and DAR formats, and the format used in your institution, if different.

Vignette: Sally was discharged home with the twins on the evening of her third postpartal day. On the morning of day 5, she is visited by the public health nurse specializing in maternal/newborn care.

   Sally is dressed in a robe and slippers, her hair is uncombed, her color is pale, and she has dark circles under her eyes. She is sitting in a recliner, bottle feeding Baby A. The grandmother is sitting on the couch feeding Baby B. Living area is noted to be clean and neat with comfortable ambient temperature. The older two children are reported to be at preschool from 9:00 AM to 2:30 PM daily.

   Postpartal assessment form is completed with physical findings within normal limits. Sally reports her bowels are working "slowly" (small firm BM this AM) with fluid intake approximately 2 liters per day and moderate appetite—"just too tired to really eat or do anything else." Sally's mother indicates she is providing household assistance—cooking, cleaning, and child care. Sally and her mother agree fatigue is a major concern for Sally. Both Sally and her mother are up twice during the night to feed the twins. Sally does take short naps during the day. Sally is observed to display usual attachment behaviors toward Baby A (Laura); however, her interaction with Baby B (unnamed) is of short duration, appears to lack warmth, and is restricted to caretaking activities.

   You provide Sally a teaching sheet describing postpartal fatigue and discussing dietary needs/supplements, energy conservation techniques, and the importance of balanced activity/exercise and rest. You suggest Sally's husband might get up for one feeding during the night to allow her a longer period of uninterrupted sleep and provide him additional opportunity for interaction with his daughters.

   Next, you ask Sally how she feels about being the mother of twins. Sally becomes tearful and states "I just don't know what I'm going to do when Mom goes home." You ask if she would like to have a visit from a member of the Mother's of Multiples group. You also suggest having a family meeting to problem-solve her concerns. You then discuss your observation that Sally appears more comfortable with Laura than with her twin, asking Sally to describe her perceptions of and feelings for Baby B. After reflecting on the question, Sally says she has felt so overwhelmed that she hasn't truly accepted the reality of having twins. She is visibly upset, berating herself for being a "poor mother." You tell her that it is not unusual to be overwhelmed by the reality of a multiple birth, even when planned for in advance of delivery.

   You ask Sally to think about what she needs to help her resolve this situation. Sally decides she needs to spend more time getting to know Baby "B", allowing other family members to care for and interact with Laura. Following a discussion about the individual characteristics of her other children, Sally says Baby "B" is unique in her level of alertness and her "acceptance" of anyone who cares for her. "She deserves a name reflecting family ties and thanksgiving for the special gift of twins." You encourage Sally to read the literature about twins provided prior to her discharge and to apply techniques she has found successful in dealing with previous stressful situations. You schedule a follow-up visit for 1 week and leave a contact number if Sally has any questions or needs assistance before your next visit. When you depart, Sally appears focused on ways to improve her current situation—smiling, displaying a lighter mood, and giving a firm handshake.

POMR/SOAP FORMAT: Problem: _____

S: _____

_____

O: _____

_____

A: _____

_____

P: _____

_____

I: _____

_____

E: _____

_____

R: _____

_____

DAR FORMAT: Focus: _____

D: _____

_____

_____

_____

A: _____

_____

_____

_____

R: _____

_____

_____

_____

FORMAT USED IN YOUR INSTITUTION/AGENCY, if different:

_____

_____

_____

_____

_____

BIBLIOGRAPHY

Fischbach, F.T. (1991). *Documenting Care: Communication, the Nursing Process and Documentation Standards.* Philadelphia: F.A. Davis.

Kerr, S.D. (1992). A comparison of four nursing documentation systems. *Journal of Nursing Staff Development, 8*(1):26–31.

Lampe, S.S. (1988). Focus Charting™. Minneapolis: Creative Nursing Management.

Yocum, F. (1993). *Documentation Skills for Quality Patient Care.* Tipp City, OH: Awareness Productions.

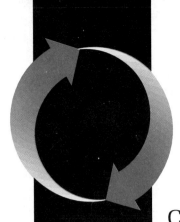

CHAPTER 8

Interactive Care Planning: From Assessment to Patient Response

This final chapter provides you the opportunity to apply and evaluate the steps of the nursing process presented in the previous chapters. A case study based on simulated assessment data gathered on your patient, Mr. Simmons, and the inclusion of physician admission orders add to the realism of this nursing process exercise. The objective and subjective data are organized within the Doenges and Moorhouse 13 diagnostic divisions assessment tool, which was described earlier in Chapter 2. (A copy of the complete assessment tool is available for your future use in Appendix B.)

INSTRUCTIONS FOR CASE STUDY

First, read over the admitting physician's orders and reflect on how your implementation of these orders will assist you in structuring Mr. Simmons' plan of care. After reviewing the physician's orders, review the extensive patient data base gathered on Mr. Simmons. As you study the data base, start to record or highlight those subjective and objective cues that suggest a problem or need and may be similar to the defining characteristics of possible nursing diagnoses for Mr. Simmons.

One purpose of this exercise is for you to identify two accurate nursing diagnoses. The accuracy of your nursing diagnoses depends on the availability of the subjective and objective data that was gathered during the admission history and physical examination and the subsequent matching of these data with the defining characteristics of the nursing diagnoses described by NANDA. Remember, all the NANDA nursing diagnoses, their related/risk factors, and defining characteristics are included in Appendix A.

To further assist you in comparing Mr. Simmons' assessment data with the defining characteristics of possible nursing diagnoses, Table 8–1 presents the 13 diagnostic divisions with selected associated NANDA nursing diagnoses. By reviewing this information, you will be able to better visualize the relationship between the varied nursing diagnoses and the focused assessments of the different diagnostic divisions.

For example, when analyzing the patient's assessment data gathered in the ELIMINATION diagnostic division, if abnormal subjective and/or objective data are present, your next step would be to direct your attention to Table 8–1. Review the 12 NANDA nursing diagnoses associated with the Elimination diagnostic division. To help you in this analysis, Box 8–1 (see page 156) displays the diagnostic division of Elimination and the 12 associated nursing diagnoses. Once you have identified a possible nursing diagnosis from the Elimination division, your next task is to review the defining characteristics of that nursing diagnosis (Appendix A) and determine if there is an accurate match with your data. Box 8–2 (see page 156) provides an abbreviated checklist to assist you as you begin diagnosing and constructing plans of care.

CASE STUDY CARE PLANNING WORKSHEET

Use the case study care planning worksheets on pages 167 to 174 to enter your two patient diagnostic statements (NANDA nursing diagnosis label, the related factors [etiologies], and evidence of signs/symptoms you used in making the diagnosis) for Mr. Simmons. Then use the worksheets to list two outcome statements for each of the diagnostic statements you have identified for Mr. Simmons. Next, select at least three nursing interventions that will assist Mr. Simmons in achieving the two measurable outcome statements you have listed and record them in the space provided on the worksheets.

The two-page Interactive Care Plan Worksheet described can also assist you during this care planning and evaluation exercise. Review the TIME OUT sections to further assist you in accurately complying with the criteria required for developing accurate diagnostic statements, constructing patient outcome statements, and in selecting appropriate nursing interventions.

CARE PLANNING EVALUATION CHECKLIST

The evaluation checklist (Fig. 8–1; see page 158) is included in this chapter to provide a workable guide for constructing Mr. Simmons' plan of care as well as future care planning assignments. The evaluation checklist was de-

Table 8–1 NURSING DIAGNOSES ORGANIZED ACCORDING TO DIAGNOSTIC DIVISIONS

After data have been collected and areas of concern/need have been identified, consult the Diagnostic Divisions framework to review the list of nursing diagnoses that fall within the individual categories. This will assist you with the choice of the specific diagnostic labels to accurately describe the data from the patient data base. Then, with the addition of etiology (when known) and signs and symptoms, the patient diagnostic statement emerges.

Diagnostic Division: Activity/Rest: Ability to engage in necessary/desired activities of life (work and leisure) and to obtain adequate sleep/rest

Diagnoses

Activity Intolerance [specify level]
Activity Intolerance, risk
Disuse Syndrome, risk for
Diversional Activity deficit
Fatigue
Sleep Pattern disturbance

Diagnostic Division: Circulation: Ability to transport oxygen and nutrients necessary to meet cellular needs

Diagnoses

Adaptive Capacity: Intracranial, decreased
Cardiac Output, decreased
Dysreflexia
Tissue Perfusion, altered, (specify): cerebral, cardiopulmonary, renal, gastrointestinal, peripheral

Diagnostic Division: Ego Integrity: Ability to develop and use skills and behaviors to integrate and manage life experiences

Diagnoses

Adjustment, impaired
Anxiety [specify level]
Body Image disturbance
Coping, defensive
Coping, Individual, ineffective
Decisional Conflict (specify)
Denial, ineffective
Energy Field, disturbance
Fear
Grieving, anticipatory
Grieving, dysfunctional
Hopelessness
Loneliness, risk for
Personal Identity disturbance
Post-Trauma Response
Powerlessness
Rape-Trauma Syndrome
Rape-Trauma Syndrome: compound reaction
Rape-Trauma Syndrome: silent reaction
Relocation Stress Syndrome
Self Esteem, chronic low
Self Esteem, disturbance
Self Esteem, situational low
Spiritual Distress
Spiritual Well Being, potential for enhancement

Diagnostic Division: Elimination: Ability to excrete waste products

Diagnoses

Bowel Incontinence
Constipation

(Continued)

Diagnoses
Constipation,colonic
Constipation, perceived
Diarrhea
Incontinence, functional
Incontinence, reflex
Incontinence, stress
Incontinence, total
Incontinence, urge
Urinary Elmination, altered patterns
Urinary Retention [acute/chronic]

Diagnostic Division: Food/Fluid: Ability to maintain intake of and utilize nutrients and liquids to meet physiologic needs
Diagnoses
Breastfeeding, effective
Breastfeeding, ineffective
Breastfeeding, interrupted
Fluid Volume deficit [active loss]
Fluid Volume deficit [regulatory failure]
Fluid Volume deficit, risk for
Fluid Volume excess
Infant Feeding Pattern, ineffective
Nutrition, altered, less than body requirements
Nutrition, altered, more than body requirements
Nutrition, altered, risk for more than body requirements
Oral Mucous Membranes, altered
Swallowing, impaired

Diagnostic Division: Hygiene: Ability to perform activities of daily living
Diagnoses
Self Care deficit (specify): feeding, bathing/hygiene, dressing/grooming, toileting

Diagnostic Division: Neurosensory: Ability to perceive, integrate, and respond to internal and external cues
Diagnoses
Confusion, acute
Confusion, chronic
Infant Behavior: disorganized
Infant Behavior: disorganized, risk for
Infant Behavior: organized
Memory, impaired
Peripheral Neurovascular dysfunction, risk for
Sensory-Perceptual alterations (specify): visual, auditory, kinesthetic, gustatory, tactile, olfactory
Thought Processes, altered
Unilateral Neglect

Diagnostic Division: Pain/Discomfort: Ability to control internal/external environment to maintain comfort
Diagnoses
Pain [acute]
Pain, chronic

Diagnostic Division: Respiration: Ability to provide and use oxygen to meet physiologic needs
Diagnoses
Airway Clearance, ineffective
Aspiration, risk for
Breathing Pattern, ineffective
Gas Exchange, impaired
Spontaneous Ventilation, inability to sustain
Ventilatory Weaning Response, dysfunctional (DVWR)

(Continued)

Table 8–1 NURSING DIAGNOSES ORGANIZED ACCORDING TO DIAGNOSTIC DIVISIONS (Continued)

Diagostic Division: Safety: Ability to provide safe, growth promoting environment

Diagnoses

Body Temperature, altered, risk for
Environmental Interpretation Syndrome, impaired
Health Maintenance, altered
Home Maintenance Management, impaired
Hyperthermia
Hypothermia
Infection, risk for
Injury, risk for
Perioperative Positioning Injury, risk for
Physical Mobility, impaired
Poisoning, risk for
Protection, altered
Self-Multilation, risk for
Skin Integrity, impaired
Skin Integrity, impaired, risk for
Suffocation, risk for
Thermoregulation, ineffective
Tissue Integrity, impaired
Trauma, risk for
Violence, risk for, directed at self/others

Diagnostic Division: Sexuality: [Component of Ego Integrity and Social Interaction] Ability to meet requirements/characteristics of male/female role

Diagnoses

Sexual Dysfunction
Sexuality Patterns, altered

Diagnostic Division: Social Interaction: Ability to establish and maintain relationships

Diagnoses

Caregiver Role Strain
Caregiver Role Strain, risk for
Communication, impaired, verbal
Community Coping, ineffective
Community Coping, potential for enhancement
Family Coping, ineffective: compromised
Family Coping, ineffective: disabling
Family Coping: potential for growth
Family Process, altered: alcoholism
Family Processes, altered
Parent/Infant/Child Attachment, altered, risk for
Parenting, altered
Parenting, altered, risk for
Role Performance, altered
Social Interaction, impaired
Social Isolation

Diagnostic Division: Teaching/Learning: Ability to incorporate and use information to achieve healthy lifestyle/optimal wellness

Diagnoses

Growth and Development, altered
Health-Seeking Behaviors (specify)
Knowledge deficit [Learning need] (specify)
Noncompliance [Compliance, altered] (specify)
Therapeutic Regimen: Community, ineffective management
Therapeutic Regimen: Families, ineffective management
Therapeutic Regimen: Individual, effective management
Therapeutic Regimen (Individual), ineffective management of

BOX 8–1　ELIMINATION DIAGNOSTIC DIVISION AND NURSING DIAGNOSES

Elimination: ability to excrete waste products

Associated Nursing Diagnoses

Bowel Incontinence
Constipation
Constipation, colonic
Constipation, perceived
Diarrhea
Incontinence, functional
Incontinence, reflex
Incontinence, stress
Incontinence, total
Incontinence, urge
Urinary Elimination, altered
Urinary Retention [acute/chronic]

BOX 8–2　DIAGNOSTIC DECISION MAKING

1. Read the physician's admitting orders.
2. Review all of the data included in the 13 diagnostic divisions. Pay particular attention to Mr. Simmons' subjective data, which describes his perception of his illness and his responses to the various health-care problems described.
3. Review the discharge considerations section at the end of the assessment tool. Can this information assist you in accurately identifying his nursing diagnoses?
4. Record or highlight any abnormal responses or observations identified while reviewing Mr. Simmons' assessment data.
5. Review the assessment tool's individual diagnostic divisions where you recorded or highlighted abnormal data.
6. In those divisions where abnormal data were highlighted, review the nursing diagnoses associated with the diagnostic division (see Table 8–1).
7. Select a possible nursing diagnosis from the diagnostic division.
8. Review the defining characteristics of your selected possible nursing diagnosis (see Appendix A).
9. Compare the recorded or highlighted data with the selected nursing diagnosis' defining characteristics. Is there sufficient match? _____ (refer to Appendix E, Lunney's Scale.) "Yes": move to step 10. "No": return to the assessment tool and ensure you have reviewed all the appropriate data. If your review is sufficient, then return to step 6 as another possible nursing diagnosis may be appropriate for consideration.

(Continued)

BOX 8–2   DIAGNOSTIC DECISION MAKING (Continued)

10. Once you have decided on an accurate nursing diagnosis complete the patient diagnostic statement by adding the related factor(s) specific to Mr. Simmons' situation (refer again to Appendix A).

11. Now develop a patient outcome statement for Mr. Simmons' identified nursing diagnosis. Two options are available for this step.
    a. Look at the nursing diagnosis and define how Mr. Simmons could resolve this identified response to his health care problem. For example, if his nursing diagnosis is Anxiety, an appropriate path in the development of an outcome statement would include "a reduction or elimination of his identified anxiety."
    b. A second strategy in outcome statement development is to review the *related factor(s)* and develop an outcome reflecting either elimination or reduction of the related factor(s). For example, if the Anxiety is determined to be related to a change in health status, then his outcome statement could reflect a correction in health status or return to premorbid state, or in this case, more appropriately, an increase in Mr. Simmons' control of his condition.

12. Once you have developed the outcome statements for Mr. Simmons, your attention must now turn to selecting appropriate nursing interventions to assist him in achieving the desired outcome. Several methods can be employed to assist you in selecting nursing interventions.

    For example: Your assigned medical-surgical or fundamentals texts are excellent resources for nursing interventions and their rationales. Other resources include care planning guides (such as Doenges, Moorhouse, and Geissler's *Nursing Care Plans*, 3rd ed, 1993) or nursing diagnoses handbooks (such as Doenges and Moorhouse's *Nurse's Pocket Guide*, 4th ed, 1993) that provide outcome statements and nursing interventions for each NANDA nursing diagnosis.

13. Repeat steps 6 to 12 for your second nursing diagnosis.

---

signed to include the criteria presented in the TIME OUT sections of the Interactive Care Plan worksheets, the requirements of the ANA's Standards of Clinical Nursing Practice presented in the previous chapters, and the current standards for JCAHO Management of Information. An additional copy of the checklist is included so you'll be able to take it with you to your assigned nursing unit and use it to help construct plans of care and evaluate your implementation of the steps of the nursing process.

Use the evaluation checklist after you have documented your first attempts at identifying Mr. Simmons' two nursing diagnoses, his two measurable outcome statements, and the appropriate nursing interventions for each outcome statement. Review the checklist's criteria against your completed case study care plan worksheet for feedback on how well your plan of care for Mr. Simmons is being accomplished.

	CRITERIA	Yes	No	Instructor's Comments

1.   Patient assessment data includes areas of biophysical, psychosocial, environmental, self-care, and/or discharge planning.

2.   Appropriate assessment techniques used (Interviewing, questioning).

3.   Assessment data is documented in appropriate manner (nursing history form, progress note, flow sheet).

4.   Patient diagnostic statement is accurately derived from assessment data.

5.   Patient diagnostic statement is verified against NANDA defining characteristics and related factors.

6.   Patient diagnostic statement is verified with patient, significant other(s), and/or other health care providers.

7.   Patient's desired outcome is derived from the identified diagnostic statement.

8.   Outcome is specific to the identified diagnostic statement.

9.   Outcome is realistic in relation to the patient's current and potential resources and capabilities.

10. Outcome is attainable in relation to the patient's current and potential resources and capabilities.

11. Outcome includes a realistic timeframe for attainment.

12. Outcome is mutually formulated with patient and/or significant other(s).

13. Plan of care includes nursing interventions based on the identified patient diagnostic statement and the desired outcome.

14. Selected nursing interventions assist the patient in attaining the desired outcome.

15. Interventions include monitoring of the patient's response to the implemented nursing interventions.

Figure 8–1. Evaluation checklist for interactive care plan worksheets. (Adapted in part from ANA Standards of Clinical Nursing Practice and the Joint Commission Standards for Management of Information.)

(Continued)

CRITERIA	Yes	No	Instructor's Comments

16. Interventions include monitoring of the patient's response toward the attainment of the outcome.

17. Interventions include the qualifiers of who, what, how, amount, time and frequency.

18. The action verb describing the nursing intervention focuses on the nurse's behavior not patient.

19. Interventions are implemented in a safe manner.

20. Rationale included for a selected nursing intervention thoroughly explains the reason for selection and the desired effect of implementation.

21. Reassessment is used to revise patient diagnostic statements, desired outcomes and/or nursing interventions.

22. Evaluation includes the patient's response to implemented nursing interventions.

23. Evaluation includes the patient's progress toward desired outcome attainment.

24. Documentation of patient care includes reassessment data.

25. Documentation of patient care includes reference to nursing interventions implemented.

26. Documentation of patient care includes reference to the patient's response to nursing interventions.

Figure 8–1. Continued

CONCLUSION

The nursing process steps described in this text are an integral part of the day-to-day science and practice of nursing. Regardless of the nursing practice setting you choose, the steps of the nursing process are universal in their application.

It is our hope that this interactive approach was helpful in learning and using the steps of the nursing process. The several interactive approaches were all designed to assist in your development of the necessary cognitive, affective, and psychomotor learning skills required to successfully apply the decision-making steps used in the nursing process. We extend our best wishes to you as you begin your nursing career.

PUTTING TOGETHER WHAT YOU HAVE LEARNED ABOUT THE NURSING PROCESS

Review the following vignette and nursing history. Then, create a plan of care for your patient, Mr. Simmons. Identify two patient problems/needs and write the patient diagnostic statement and two outcomes. Choose three interventions for each patient diagnostic statement.

Vignette: Mr. R. Simmons, who has had non–insulin-dependent diabetes mellitus (NIDDM) for 5 years, presented to his physician's office with a nonhealing ulcer on his left foot, of 3 weeks' duration. Laboratory studies at that time revealed blood glucose of 256 per finger stick and urine dipstick—ketones small.

Admitting Physician's Orders

Culture/sensitivity and Gram's stain of foot ulcer
Random blood glucose on admission and finger stick BG every AM
CBC, electrolytes, glycosylated Hb in AM
Chest x-ray & ECG in AM
NPH insulin 15 U q AM. Begin insulin instruction for postdischarge self-
   care
Dicloxacillin 500 mg po q 6 hr; start after culture obtained
Darvon 65 mg q 4 hr prn for pain
Diet–2400 calories ADA/three meals with two snacks
Up in chair ad lib with feet elevated
Foot cradle for bed
Betadine soak L foot tid × 15 min, then cover with dry sterile dressing
Vital signs qid

Patient Assessment Data Base

Name: R. Simmons   **Informant:** Patient
Reliability (Scale 1–4): 3
Age: 67   **DOB:** 5/3/27   **Race:** Caucasian   **Sex:** M
Adm. date: 6/28/94   **Time:** 7 PM   **From:** Home

ACTIVITY/REST

Reports (Subjective)

Occupation: Farmer
Usual activities/hobbies: reading, playing cards. "Don't have time to do much. Anyway I'm too tired most of the time to do anything after the chores."
Limitations imposed by illness: "I have to watch what I order if I eat out."
Sleep: Hours: 6–8 hrs/night   **Naps:** no   **Aids:** no
Insomnia: "not unless I drink coffee after supper." Usually feels rested when awakens at 4:30 AM.

Exhibits (Objective)

Observed response to activity: favors L foot when walking
Mental status: alert/active
Neuro/muscular assessment: muscle mass/tone: bilaterally equal/firm
  Posture: erect   **ROM**: full
  Strength: equal three extremities/favors L foot currently

CIRCULATION

Reports (Subjective)

History of slow healing: lesion L foot, 3 weeks.
Extremities: numbness/tingling: "My feet feel cold and tingling when I walk a lot."
Cough/character of sputum: occ./white
Change in frequency/amount of urine: yes/voiding more lately

Exhibits (Objective)

Peripheral pulses: radials 31; popliteal, dorsalis, postibial/pedal, all 1+
B/P: R: Sit: 140/86   **Lying:** 146/90   **Stand:** 138/90
  L: Sit: 138/88   **Lying:** 142/88   **Stand:** 138/84
Pulse: Apical: 86 **Radial:** 86 **Quality:** strong   **Rhythm:** regular
Chest auscultation: few wheezes clear with cough, no murmurs/rubs
Jugular vein distention: -0-
Extremities:
  Temperature: feet cool bilat./legs warm
  Color: skin: legs pale
  Capillary refill: slow both feet
  Homan's sign: -0- **Varicosities:** few enlarged superficial veins both calves
  Nails: toenails thickened, yellow, brittle
  Distribution and quality of hair: coarse hair to midcalf, none on ankles/toes
Color: General: ruddy face/arms   **Mucous membranes/lips:** pink
  Nail beds: blanch well   **Conjunctiva and sclera:** white

EGO INTEGRITY

Reports (Subjective)

Report of stress factors: "normal farmer's problems: weather, pests, bankers, etc."
Ways of handling stress: "I get busy with the chores and talk things over with my livestock, they listen pretty good."
Financial concerns: no insurance, needs to hire someone while here.
Relationship status: married   **Cultural factors:** rural/agrarian, eastern European descent
Religion: Protestant/practicing
Lifestyle: middle class/self-sufficient farmer
Recent changes: no
Feelings: "I'm in control of most things, except this diabetes now." Concerned re possible therapy change "from pills to shots."

Exhibits (Objective)

Emotional status: calm most of time
Observed physiologic response(s): occasionally sighs deeply/frowns, shrugs shoulders/throws up hands, appears frustrated

ELIMINATION

Reports (Subjective)

Usual bowel pattern: most every PM
Last BM: last night   **Character of stool:** firm/brown
Bleeding: -0-   **Hemorrhoids:** -0-   **Constipation:** occ.
Laxative used: hot prune juice
Urinary: no problems   **Character of urine:** pale yellow

Exhibits (Objective)

Abd. tender: no   **Soft/firm:** soft   **Palpable mass:** none
Bowel sounds: active all four quads

FOOD/FLUID

Reports (Subjective)

Usual diet (type): 2400 ADA (occ. "cheats" with dessert, "My wife watches it pretty closely.")
No. of meals daily: 3/1 snack
Dietary pattern:
  B: fruit juice/toast/ham/coffee
  L: meat/potatoes/veg/fruit/milk
  D: meat sandwich/soup/fruit/coffee
  Snack: milk/crackers at hs.   **Usual beverage:** skim milk, 2–3 cups decaf coffee, and drinks lots of water.
Last meal/intake: Dinner: roast beef sandwich, vegetable soup, pear with cheese, decaf
Loss of appetite: "Never, but lately I don't feel as hungry as usual."
Nausea/vomiting: -0-   **Food allergies:** none
Heartburn/food intolerance: cabbage causes gas, coffee after supper causes heartburn.
Mastication/swallowing probs: No   **Dentures:** partial upper plate
Usual weight: 175   **Recent changes:** has lost about 3 lbs this month.
Diuretic therapy: no

Exhibits (Objective)

Wt: 171 lb   **Ht:** 59100   **Build:** stocky   **Skin turgor:** good/leathery
Appearance of tongue: midline, pink   **Mucous membranes:** pink, intact
Condition of teeth/gums: good, no irritation/bleeding noted
Breath sounds: few wheezes cleared with cough
Bowel sounds: active all four quads

HYGIENE

Reports (Subjective)

Activities of daily living: independent in all areas
Preferred time of bath: PM

Exhibits (Objective)

General appearance: clean, shaven, short cut hair, hands rough and dry
Scalp & eyebrows: scaly white patches

NEUROSENSORY

Reports (Subjective)

Headache: "Occasionally behind my eyes when I worry too much."
Tingling/Numbness: feet, occasionally

Eyes: vision loss; far-sighted   **Exam:** 2 yr ago
Ears: Hearing loss   **R:** "some"   **L:** no (has not been tested)
Nose: Epistaxis: -0-   **Sense of smell:** states no problem

Exhibits (Objective)

Mental status: alert; oriented to time, place, person
Affect: concerned   **Memory: Remote/Recent:** clear and intact
Speech: clear/coherent
Pupil reaction: PERLA/small   **Glasses:** reading   **Hearing Aid:** no
Handgrip/release: strong/equal

PAIN/DISCOMFORT

Reports (Subjective)

Location: L foot   **Intensity (1–10):** 5–6   **Quality:** dull ache with occ. sharp stabbing
Frequency/duration: "Seems like all the time."   **Radiation:** no
Precipitating factors: shoes, walking   **How relieved:** ASA, not helping
Other complaints: sometimes has back pain following chores/heavy lifting, relieved by ASA/ liniment rubdown.

Exhibits (Objective)

Facial grimacing: when lesion border palpated
Guarding affected area: pulls foot away   **Narrowed focus:** no
Emotional response: tense, irritated

RESPIRATION

Reports (Subjective)

Dyspnea: -0-   **Cough:** occ. morning cough, white sputum
Emphysema: -0-   **Bronchitis:** -0-   **Asthma:** -0-   **Tuberculosis:** -0-
Smoker: filters   **Pack/day:** 1/2 **No. of pack years**: 251
Use of respiratory aids: -0-

Exhibits (Objective)

Respiratory rate: 22   **Depth:** good   **Symmetry:** equal, bilateral
Auscultation: few wheezes, clear with cough
Cyanosis: -0-   **Clubbing of fingers:** -0-
Sputum characteristics: none to observe
Mentation/restlessness: alert/oriented/relaxed

SAFETY

Reports (Subjective)

Allergies: -0-   **Blood transfusions:** -0-
Sexually transmitted disease: none
Fractures/dislocations: L clavicle, 1962, fell getting off tractor
Arthritis/unstable joints: "I think I've got some in my knees."
Back problems: occ. lower back pain
Vision impaired: requires glasses for reading
Hearing impaired: slightly (R), compensates by turning "good ear" toward speaker

Exhibits (Objective)

Temperature: 99.4°F oral
Skin integrity: impaired L foot   **Scars:** R inguinal, surgical

Rashes: -0-   **Bruises:** -0-   **Lacerations**: -0-   **Blisters:** -0-
Ulcerations: medial aspect L foot, 2.5 cm diameter, approx. 3 mm deep, draining sm. amt. cream color/pink-tinged matter, no odor noted
Strength (general): equal all extremities   **Muscle tone:** firm
ROM: good   **Gait:** favors L foot   **Paresthesia/Paralysis:** -0-

SEXUALITY: MALE

Reports (Subjective)

Penile discharge: -0-   **Prostate disorder:** -0-   **Vasectomy:** -0-
Last proctoscopic exam: 2 yr ago.   **Prostate exam:** 1 yr ago
Practice self-exam: Breast/testicles: No
Problems/complaints: "I don't have any problems, but you'd have to ask my wife if there are any complaints."
Exhibits (Objective)
Exam: Breast: no masses   **Testicles:** deferred   **Prostate:** deferred

SOCIAL INTERACTIONS

Reports (Subjective)

Marital status: married 43 yr   **Living with:** wife
Report of problems: none
Extended family: one daughter lives in town (30 miles away); one daughter married/grandson, living out of state
Other: several couples, he & wife play cards/socialize with 2–3 times/month
Role: works farm alone; husband/father/grandfather
Report of problems related to illness/condition: none until now
Coping behaviors: "My wife and I have always talked things out.
You know the 11th commandment is 'Thou shalt not go to bed angry.'"

Exhibits (Objective)

Speech: clear, intelligible
Verbal/nonverbal communication with family/SO(s): speaks quietly with wife, looking her in the eye; relaxed posture
Family interaction patterns: wife sitting at bedside, relaxed, both reading paper, making occasional comments to each other

TEACHING/LEARNING

Reports (Subjective)

Dominant language: English   **Literate:** Yes
Education level: 2 yr college
Health beliefs/practices: "I take care of the minor problems and only see the doctor when something's broken."
Familial risk factors/relationship:
  Diabetes: Uncle   **Tuberculosis:** brother died, age 27
  Heart Disease: f. died, age 78, heart attack
  Strokes: mo. died, age 81   **High B/P:** mo.
Prescribed medications:
  Drug: Orinase   **Dose:** 250 mg   **Schedule:** 8 AM/6 PM, Last dose 6 PM today   **Purpose:** control diabetes
Home glucose monitoring: "Stopped several months ago when I ran out of TesTape. It was always negative anyway."
Does patient take medications regularly? yes

Nonprescription (OTC) drugs: occ. ASA
Use of alcohol (amount/frequency): socially, occ. beer
Tobacco: 1/2 pack/day
Admitting diagnosis (physician): hyperglycemia and lesion L foot
Reason for hospitalization (patient): "Sore on foot & my sugar is up."
History of current complaint: "Three weeks ago I got a blister on my foot from breaking in my new boots. It got sore so I lanced it, but it isn't getting any better."
Patient's expectations of this hospitalization: "Clear up this infection and control my diabetes."
Other relevant illness &/or previous hospitalizations/surgeries: 1965 R inguinal hernia repair
Evidence of failure to improve: lesion L foot, 3 wk
Last physical exam: complete 1 yr ago, office follow-up 3 mo ago

Discharge Considerations (as of 6/28)

Anticipated discharge: 7/1/94 (3 days)
Resources: self; wife
Financial: "If this doesn't take too long to heal, we got some savings to cover things."
Anticipated lifestyle changes: none
Assistance needed: may require farm help for several days
Teaching: learn new medication regimen and wound care; review diet
Community Supports: Diabetic Support Group
Referral: Supplies: Downtown Pharmacy or AARP
        Equipment: Glucometer—AARP

INTERACTIVE CARE PLAN WORKSHEET

Student Name:

Patient's Medical Diagnosis:

NURSING DIAGNOSIS

DEFINITION:

DEFINING CHARACTERISTICS:

RELATED FACTORS:

STUDENT INSTRUCTIONS: In the space below enter the subjective and objective data gathered during your patient assessment.

Subjective Data Entry

Objective Data Entry

A S S E S S M E N T

TIME OUT!

Student Instructions: To be sure your patient diagnostic statement written below is accurate, you need to review the defining characteristics and related factors associated with the nursing diagnosis and see how your patient data matches. Do you have an accurate match or is additional data required or does another nursing diagnosis need to be investigated?

PATIENT DIAGNOSTIC STATEMENT:

D I A G N O S I S

Nursing Diagnosis (specify) _____

Related to _____

© 1993 F.A. Davis

167

PLANNING

Desired Outcome and Patient Criteria: The Patient will:

TIME OUT! The desired outcome must meet criteria to be accurate. The outcome must be specific, realistic, measurable, and include a time frame for completion. Does the action verb describe the patient's behavior to be evaluated? Can the outcome be used in the evaluation step of the nursing process to measure the patient's response to the nursing interventions listed below?

Interventions	Rationale for Selected Intervention and References

EVALUATION

TIME OUT! Do your interventions assist in achieving the desired outcome? Do your interventions address further monitoring of the patient's response to your interventions and to the achievement of the desired outcome? Are qualifiers: **when, how, amount, time,** and **frequency** used? Is the focus of the action's verb on the nurse's actions and not on the patient? Do your rationales provide sufficient reason and directions?

What was your patient's response to the interventions?

Was the desired outcome achieved? If no, what revisions to either the desired outcome or interventions would you make?
☐ Yes ☐ No

DOCUMENTATION

Documentation Focus: Now that you have completed the evaluation, the next step is to document your care and the patient's response. Use the areas below to enter your progress note information.

Reassessment Data:

Interventions Implemented:

Patient's Response:

INSTRUCTOR'S COMMENTS:

INTERACTIVE CARE PLAN WORKSHEET

Student Name:

Patient's Medical Diagnosis:

NURSING DIAGNOSIS

DEFINITION:

DEFINING CHARACTERISTICS:

RELATED FACTORS:

STUDENT INSTRUCTIONS:

In the space below enter the subjective and objective data gathered during your patient assessment.

Subjective Data Entry

Objective Data Entry

A S S E S S M E N T

TIME OUT!

Student Instructions: To be sure your patient diagnostic statement written below is accurate, you need to review the defining characteristics and related factors associated with the nursing diagnosis and see how your patient data matches. Do you have an accurate match or is additional data required or does another nursing diagnosis need to be investigated?

PATIENT DIAGNOSTIC STATEMENT:

D I A G N O S I S

Nursing Diagnosis (specify) _____

Related to _____

_____

_____

© 1993 F.A. Davis

169

PLANNING

Desired Outcome and Patient Criteria: The Patient will:

TIME OUT! The desired outcome must meet criteria to be accurate. The outcome must be specific, realistic, measurable, and include a time frame for completion. Does the action verb describe the patient's behavior to be evaluated? Can the outcome be used in the evaluation step of the nursing process to measure the patient's response to the nursing interventions listed below?

Interventions	Rationale for Selected Intervention and References

EVALUATION

TIME OUT! Do your interventions assist in achieving the desired outcome? Do your interventions address further monitoring of the patient's response to your interventions and to the achievement of the desired outcome? Are qualifiers: **when, how, amount, time,** and **frequency** used? Is the focus of the action's verb on the nurse's actions and not on the patient? Do your rationales provide sufficient reason and directions?

What was your patient's response to the interventions?

Was the desired outcome achieved?   If no, what revisions to either the desired outcome or interventions would you make?
☐ Yes ☐ No

DOCUMENTATION

Documentation Focus: Now that you have completed the evaluation, the next step is to document your care and the patient's response. Use the areas below to enter your progress note information.

Reassessment Data:

Interventions Implemented:

Patient's Response:

INSTRUCTOR'S COMMENTS:

INTERACTIVE CARE PLAN WORKSHEET

Student Name:

Patient's Medical Diagnosis:

NURSING DIAGNOSIS

DEFINITION:

DEFINING CHARACTERISTICS:

RELATED FACTORS:

STUDENT INSTRUCTIONS:

In the space below enter the subjective and objective data gathered during your patient assessment.

Subjective Data Entry

Objective Data Entry

A S S E S S M E N T

TIME OUT!

Student Instructions: To be sure your patient diagnostic statement written below is accurate, you need to review the defining characteristics and related factors associated with the nursing diagnosis and see how your patient data matches. Do you have an accurate match or is additional data required or does another nursing diagnosis need to be investigated?

PATIENT DIAGNOSTIC STATEMENT:

D I A G N O S I S

Nursing Diagnosis (specify) _____

Related to _____

PLANNING

Desired Outcome and Patient Criteria: The Patient will:

TIME OUT! The desired outcome must meet criteria to be accurate. The outcome must be specific, realistic, measurable, and include a time frame for completion. Does the action verb describe the patient's behavior to be evaluated? Can the outcome be used in the evaluation step of the nursing process to measure the patient's response to the nursing interventions listed below?

Interventions	Rationale for Selected Intervention and References

EVALUATION

TIME OUT! Do your interventions assist in achieving the desired outcome? Do your interventions address further monitoring of the patient's response to your interventions and to the achievement of the desired outcome? Are qualifiers: **when, how, amount, time,** and **frequency** used? Is the focus of the action's verb on the nurse's actions and not on the patient? Do your rationales provide sufficient reason and directions?

What was your patient's response to the interventions?

Was the desired outcome achieved?   If no, what revisions to either the desired outcome or interventions would you make?
☐ Yes   ☐ No

DOCUMENTATION

Documentation Focus: Now that you have completed the evaluation, the next step is to document your care and the patient's response. Use the areas below to enter your progress note information.

Reassessment Data:

Interventions Implemented:

Patient's Response:

INSTRUCTOR'S COMMENTS:

INTERACTIVE CARE PLAN WORKSHEET

Student Name:

Patient's Medical Diagnosis:

NURSING DIAGNOSIS

DEFINITION:

DEFINING CHARACTERISTICS:

RELATED FACTORS:

STUDENT INSTRUCTIONS: In the space below enter the subjective and objective data gathered during your patient assessment.

Subjective Data Entry

Objective Data Entry

A S S E S S M E N T

TIME OUT!

Student Instructions: To be sure your patient diagnostic statement written below is accurate, you need to review the defining characteristics and related factors associated with the nursing diagnosis and see how your patient data matches. Do you have an accurate match or is additional data required or does another nursing diagnosis need to be investigated?

PATIENT DIAGNOSTIC STATEMENT:

D I A G N O S I S

Nursing Diagnosis (specify)

Related to

© 1993 F.A. Davis

173

PLANNING

Desired Outcome and Patient Criteria: The Patient will:

TIME OUT! The desired outcome must meet criteria to be accurate. The outcome must be specific, realistic, measurable, and include a time frame for completion. Does the action verb describe the patient's behavior to be evaluated? Can the outcome be used in the evaluation step of the nursing process to measure the patient's response to the nursing interventions listed below?

Interventions	Rationale for Selected Intervention and References

EVALUATION

TIME OUT! Do your interventions assist in achieving the desired outcome? Do your interventions address further monitoring of the patient's response to your interventions and to the achievement of the desired outcome? Are qualifiers: **when**, **how**, **amount**, **time**, and **frequency** used? Is the focus of the action's verb on the nurse's actions and not on the patient? Do your rationales provide sufficient reason and directions?

What was your patient's response to the interventions?

Was the desired outcome achieved?   If no, what revisions to either the desired outcome or interventions would you make?
☐ Yes   ☐ No

DOCUMENTATION

Documentation Focus: Now that you have completed the evaluation, the next step is to document your care and the patient's response. Use the areas below to enter your progress note information.

Reassessment Data:

Interventions Implemented:

Patient's Response:

INSTRUCTOR'S COMMENTS:

	CRITERIA	Yes	No	Instructor's Comments

1. Patient assessment data includes areas of biophysical, psychosocial, environmental, self-care, and/or discharge planning.

2. Appropriate assessment techniques used (Interviewing, questioning).

3. Assessment data is documented in appropriate manner (nursing history form, progress note, flow sheet).

4. Patient diagnostic statement is accurately derived from assessment data.

5. Patient diagnostic statement is verified against NANDA defining characteristics and related factors.

6. Patient diagnostic statement is verified with patient, significant other(s), and/or other health care providers.

7. Patient's desired outcome is derived from the identified diagnostic statement.

8. Outcome is specific to the identified diagnostic statement.

9. Outcome is realistic in relation to the patient's current and potential resources and capabilities.

10. Outcome is attainable in relation to the patient's current and potential resources and capabilities.

11. Outcome includes a realistic timeframe for attainment.

12. Outcome is mutually formulated with patient and/or significant other(s).

13. Plan of care includes nursing interventions based on the identified patient diagnostic statement and the desired outcome.

14. Selected nursing interventions assist the patient in attaining the desired outcome.

15. Interventions include monitoring of the patient's response to the implemented nursing interventions.

(*Continued*)

CRITERIA	Yes	No	Instructor's Comments

16.   Interventions include monitoring of the patient's response toward the attainment of the outcome.

17.   Interventions include the qualifiers of wno, what, how, amount, time and frequency.

18.   The action verb describing the nursing intervention focuses on the nurse's behavior not patient.

19.   Interventions are implemented in a safe manner.

20.   Rationale included for a selected nursing intervention thoroughly explains the reason for selection and the desired effect of implementation.

21.   Reassessment is used to revise patient diagnostic statements, desired outcomes and/or nursing interventions.

22.   Evaluation includes the patient's response to implemented nursing interventions.

23.   Evaluation includes the patient's progress toward desired outcome attainment.

24.   Documentation of patient care includes reassessment data.

25.   Documentation of patient care includes reference to nursing interventions implemented.

26.   Documentation of patient care includes reference to the patient's response to nursing interventions.

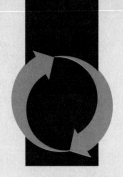

North American Nursing Diagnosis Association (NANDA) Nursing Diagnoses with Definitions, Related/ Risk Factors, and Defining Characteristics

Activity Intolerance [specify level]

DEFINITION: A state in which an individual has insufficient physiological or psychological energy to endure or complete required or desired daily activities.

RELATED FACTORS: ○ Generalized weakness ○ Sedentary lifestyle ○ Bedrest or immobility ○ Imbalance between oxygen supply and demand ○ [Cognitive deficits/emotional status; underlying disease process/depression]

DEFINING CHARACTERISTICS

SUBJECTIVE: ■ Verbal report of fatigue or weakness ○ Exertional discomfort or dyspnea ○ [Pain] ○ [Verbalizes no desire and/or lack of interest in activity]

OBJECTIVE: ○ Abnormal heart rate or blood pressure response ○ Electrocardiographic changes reflecting arrhythmias or ischemia ○ [Pallor] ○ [Cyanosis]
Suggested levels for determining degree of impairment (Gordon, 1993):

Level I: Walk, regular pace, on level indefinitely; one flight or more but more short of breath than normally

Level II: Walk one city block 500 feet on level; climb one flight slowly without stopping

---

■ = critical factors/major signs and symptoms

NOTE: Information appearing in [ ] has been added by the authors to clarify and facilitate the use of nursing diagnoses.

Level III: Walk no more than 50 feet on level without stopping; unable to climb one flight of stairs without stopping
Level IV: Dyspnea and fatigue at rest

Activity Intolerance, risk for*

DEFINITION: A state in which an individual is at risk of experiencing insufficient physiologic or psychological energy to endure or complete required or desired daily activities.

RISK FACTORS: ○ History of previous intolerance ○ Presence of circulatory/respiratory problems ○ Deconditioned status ○ Presence of circulatory/respiratory problems ○ Inexperience with the activity ○ [Early diagnosis of progressive disease state such as cancer, multiple sclerosis; extensive surgical procedures] ○ [Verbalized reluctance/inability to perform expected activity]

Adaptive Capacity: Intracranial, decreased

DEFINITION: A clinical state in which intracranial fluid dynamic mechanisms that normally compensate for increases in intracranial volumes are compromised, resulting in repeated disproportionate increases in intracranial pressure (ICP) in response to a variety of noxious and non-noxious stimuli.

RELATED FACTORS: ○ Brain injuries ○ Sustained increase in ICP greater than or equal to 10–15 mm Hg ○ Decreased cerebral perfusion pressure greater than or equal to 50–60 mm Hg ○ Systemic hypotension with intracranial hypertension

DEFINING CHARACTERISTICS

OBJECTIVE: ■ Repeated increases in ICP of greater than 10 mm Hg for more than 5 minutes following a variety of external stimuli ○ Disproportionate increase in ICP following single environmental of nursing maneuver stimulus ○ Elevated P2-ICP waveform ○ Volume pressure response test variation (Volume-pressure ratio greater than 2, Pressure-volume index less than 10) ○ Baseline ICP equal to or greater than 10 mm Hg ○ Wide amplitude ICP waveform

Adjustment, impaired

DEFINITION: The state in which the individual is unable to modify his/her lifestyle or behavior in a manner consistent with a change in health status.

RELATED FACTORS: ○ Disability requiring change in lifestyle ○ Inadequate support systems ○ Impaired cognition, sensory overload ○ Assault to self-esteem, al-

---

■ = critical factors/major signs and symptoms

NOTE: Information appearing in [ ] has been added by the authors to clarify and facilitate the use of nursing diagnoses.

*[**NOTE:** A risk diagnosis is not evidenced by signs and symptoms, since the problem has not yet occurred, and nursing interventions are directed at prevention. Therefore, risk factors present are noted instead.]

tered locus of control ○ Incomplete grieving [severe emotional loss] ○ [Physical and/or learning disability] ○ [Life-threatening condition or disease]

DEFINING CHARACTERISTICS

SUBJECTIVE: ▪ Verbalization of nonacceptance of health status change

OBJECTIVE: ▪ Nonexistent or unsuccessful ability to be involved in problem solving or goal setting ○ Lack of movement toward independence ○ Extended period of shock, disbelief, or anger regarding health status change ○ Lack of future-oriented thinking ○ [Lack of ability to limit expectations of self]

Airway Clearance, ineffective

DEFINITION: A state in which an individual is unable to clear secretions or obstructions from the respiratory tract to maintain airway patency.

RELATED FACTORS: ○ Tracheobronchial infection, obstruction, secretion ○ Decreased energy/fatigue ○ Perceptual/cognitive impairment ○ Trauma ○ [Inhalation injury]

DEFINING CHARACTERISTICS

SUBJECTIVE: ○ [Statement of difficulty breathing]

OBJECTIVE: ○ Abnormal breath sounds—rales (crackles), rhonchi (wheezes) ○ Changes in rate or depth of respiration ○ Tachypnea ○ Cough, effective or ineffective, with or without sputum ○ Cyanosis ○ Dyspnea ○ [Apnea] ○ [Fear; anxiety; restlessness] ○ [Use of accessory muscles for breathing] ○ [Choking or noisy respirations]

Anxiety [mild, moderate, severe, panic]

DEFINITION: A vague uneasy feeling whose source is often nonspecific or unknown to the individual.

RELATED FACTORS: ○ Unconscious conflict about essential values, [beliefs], and goals of life ○ Situational and [or] maturational crises ○ Interpersonal transmission/contagion ○ Threat to self-concept [perceived or actual], [unconscious conflict] ○ Threat of death [perceived or actual] ○ Threat to or change in health status [terminal illness], role functioning, environment [safety], interaction patterns, socioeconomic status ○ Unmet needs ○ [Positive or negative self-talk] ○ [Physiologic factors such as hyperthyroidism, pheochromocytoma, use of steroids]

DEFINING CHARACTERISTICS

SUBJECTIVE: ○ Increased tension ○ Regretful ○ Scared; shakiness ○ Overexcited; rattled; distressed ○ Apprehension; uncertainty; fearful ○ Feelings of inadequacy ○ Fear of unspecific consequences ○ Expressed concern regarding changes in life events ○ Worried; anxious; jittery ○ Painful and persistent increased helplessness ○ [Somatic complaints] ○ [Sleeplessness] ○ [Sense of impending doom] ○ [Hopelessness]

▪ = critical factors/major signs and symptoms

NOTE: Information appearing in [ ] has been added by the authors to clarify and facilitate the use of nursing diagnoses.

OBJECTIVE: ■ Sympathetic stimulation: cardiovascular excitation, superficial vasoconstriction, pupil dilation ○ Increased wariness; glancing about; poor eye contact ○ Extraneous movements (foot shuffling; hand/arm movements) ○ Increased perspiration ○ Trembling/hand tremors; restlessness ○ Insomnia ○ Facial tension; voice quivering ○ Focus on self ○ [Urinary frequency] ○ [Repetitive questioning] ○ [Pacing/purposeless activity] ○ [Impaired functioning/immobility]

Aspiration, risk for*

DEFINITION: The state in which an individual is at risk for entry of gastric secretions, oropharyngeal secretions, or [exogenous food] solids or fluids into tracheobronchial passages [due to dysfunction or absence of normal protective mechanisms].

RISK FACTORS: ○ Reduced level of consciousness ○ Depressed cough and gag reflexes ○ Impaired swallowing [owing to inability of the epiglottis and true vocal cords to move to close off trachea] ○ Facial/oral/neck surgery or trauma; wired jaws ○ Situation hindering elevation of upper body ○ Delayed gastric emptying; decreased gastrointestinal motility; increased intragastric pressure; increased gastric residual ○ Presence of tracheostomy or endotracheal tube; [over- or inadequate inflation of tracheostomy/endotracheal tube cuff] ○ Gastrointestinal tubes; bolus tube feedings/medication administration

Body Image disturbance

DEFINITION: Disruption in the way one perceives one's body image.

RELATED FACTORS: ○ Biophysical [physical trauma/mutilation, pregnancy, physical change caused by biochemical agents (drugs), dependence on machine] ○ Psychosocial ○ Cultural or spiritual ○ Cognitive/perceptual ○ [Significance of body part or functioning with regard to age, sex, developmental level, or basic human needs] ○ [Maturational changes]

DEFINING CHARACTERISTICS: ○ A or B must be present to justify the diagnosis of Body Image disturbance ■ A = verbal response to actual or perceived change in structure and/or function ■ B = nonverbal response to actual or perceived change in structure and/or function

The following clinical manifestations may be used to validate the presence of A or B:

SUBJECTIVE: ○ Verbalization of:

Change in lifestyle;
Fear of rejection or of reaction by others;
Focus on past strength, function, or appearance;

■ = critical factors/major signs and symptoms

NOTE: Information appearing in [ ] has been added by the authors to clarify and facilitate the use of nursing diagnoses.

*[**NOTE:** A risk diagnosis is not evidenced by signs and symptoms, since the problem has not yet occurred, and nursing interventions are directed at prevention. Therefore, risk factors present are noted instead.]

Feelings of helplessness, hopelessness, or powerlessness;
Preoccupation with change or loss;
[Feelings of depersonalization/grandiosity]

○ Refusal to verify actual change ○ Emphasis on remaining strengths, heightened achievement ○ Personalization of part or loss by name ○ Depersonalization of part or loss by impersonal pronouns ○ Extension of body boundary to incorporate environmental objects

OBJECTIVE: ○ Missing body part ○ Actual change in structure and/or function ○ Not looking at/not touching body part ○ Trauma to nonfunctioning part ○ Change in ability to estimate spatial relationship of body to environment ○ Hiding or overexposing body part (intentional or unintentional) ○ Change in social involvement ○ [Inability to differentiate internal/external stimuli/loss of ego boundaries]

Body Temperature, altered, risk for*

DEFINITION: The state in which the individual is at risk for failure to maintain body temperature within normal range.

RISK FACTORS: ○ Extremes of age, weight ○ Exposure to cold/cool or warm/hot environments ○ Dehydration ○ Inactivity or vigorous activity ○ Medications causing vasoconstriction/vasodilation, altered metabolic rate, sedation, [use or overdose of certain drugs or exposure to anesthesia] ○ Inappropriate clothing for environmental temperature ○ Illness or trauma affecting temperature regulation ○ [Infections, systemic or localized] ○ [Neoplasms, tumors, collagen/vascular disease]

Bowel Incontinence

DEFINITION: A state in which an individual experiences a change in normal bowel habits characterized by involuntary passage of stool.

RELATED FACTORS: To be developed by NANDA ○ (Neuromuscular/musculoskeletal involvement) ○ (Perceptual or cognitive impairment) ○ (Depression) ○ (Severe anxiety) ○ [Diarrhea and/or fecal impaction]
  Note: These factors were identified when this diagnosis was originally accepted and have been retained here to assist the user until NANDA completes its work.

DEFINING CHARACTERISTIC

OBJECTIVE: ■ Involuntary passage of stool

■ = critical factors/major signs and symptoms

NOTE: Information appearing in [ ] has been added by the authors to clarify and facilitate the use of nursing diagnoses.

*[**NOTE:** A risk diagnosis is not evidenced by signs and symptoms, since the problem has not yet occurred, and nursing interventions are directed at prevention. Therefore, risk factors present are noted instead.]

Breastfeeding, effective

DEFINITION: The state in which a mother-infant dyad/family exhibits adequate proficiency and satisfaction with breastfeeding process.

RELATED FACTORS: ○ Basic breastfeeding knowledge ○ Normal breast structure ○ Normal infant oral structure ○ Infant gestational age greater than 34 weeks ○ Support sources [available] ○ Maternal confidence

DEFINING CHARACTERISTICS

SUBJECTIVE: ○ Maternal verbalization of satisfaction with the breastfeeding process

OBJECTIVE: ■ Mother able to position infant at breast to promote a successful latch-on response ■ Infant is content after feedings ■ Regular and sustained sucking at the breast (8 to 10 times/24 hr) ■ Appropriate infant weight patterns [gain] for age ■ Effective mother/infant communication pattern (infant cues, maternal interpretation and response) ○ Signs and/or symptoms of oxytocin release (let down or milk ejection reflex) ○ Adequate infant elimination patterns for age [e.g., soft stools; over six wet diapers per day of unconcentrated urine]; eagerness of infant to nurse

Breastfeeding, ineffective

DEFINITION: The state in which a mother, infant, or child experiences dissatisfaction or difficulty with the breastfeeding process.

RELATED FACTORS: ○ Prematurity; infant anomaly; poor infant sucking reflex ○ Infant receiving [numerous or repeated] supplemental feedings with artificial nipple ○ Maternal anxiety or ambivalence ○ Knowledge deficit ○ Previous history of breastfeeding failure ○ Interruption in breastfeeding ○ Nonsupportive partner/family ○ Maternal breast anomaly; previous breast surgery; painful nipples/breast engorgement

DEFINING CHARACTERISTICS

SUBJECTIVE: ■ Unsatisfactory breastfeeding process ○ Persistence of sore nipples beyond the first week of breastfeeding ○ Insufficient emptying of each breast per feeding ○ Actual or perceived inadequate milk supply

OBJECTIVE: ■ Observable signs of inadequate infant intake [inappropriate weight loss/or inadequate gain, decreased urinary output] ○ [Nonsustained or] insufficient opportunity for suckling at the breast ○ Infant inability [failure] to attach on to maternal breast correctly ○ Infant arching and crying at the breasts; resisting latching on ○ Infant exhibiting fussiness and crying within the first hour after breastfeeding; unresponsive to other comfort measures ○ No observable signs of oxytocin release

---

■ = critical factors/major signs and symptoms

NOTE: Information appearing in [ ] has been added by the authors to clarify and facilitate the use of nursing diagnoses.

Breastfeeding, interrupted

DEFINITION: A break in the continuity of the breastfeeding process as a result of inability or inadvisability to put baby to breast for feeding.

RELATED FACTORS: ○ Maternal or infant illness ○ Prematurity ○ Maternal employment ○ Contraindications to breastfeeding (e.g., drugs, true breastmilk jaundice) ○ Need to abruptly wean infant

DEFINING CHARACTERISTICS

SUBJECTIVE: ■ Infant does not receive nourishment at the breast for some or all of feedings ○ Maternal desire to maintain lactation and provide (or eventually provide) her breastmilk for her infant's nutritional needs ○ Lack of knowledge regarding expression and storage of breastmilk

OBJECTIVE: ○ Separation of mother and infant

Breathing Pattern, ineffective

DEFINITION: The state in which an individual's inhalation and/or exhalation pattern does not enable adequate pulmonary inflation or emptying.

RELATED FACTORS: ○ Neuromuscular/musculoskeletal impairment ○ Anxiety ○ Pain ○ Perception/cognitive impairment ○ Decreased energy/fatigue ○ [Alteration of patient's normal O_2/CO_2 ratio, e.g., O_2 therapy in COPD]

DEFINING CHARACTERISTICS

SUBJECTIVE: ○ Shortness of breath

OBJECTIVE: ○ Dyspnea; tachypnea ○ Fremitus ○ Cough ○ Respiratory depth changes; altered chest excursion ○ Nasal flaring ○ Use of accessory muscles ○ Pursed-lip breathing/prolonged expiratory phase ○ Assumption of three-point position ○ Cyanosis; abnormal arterial blood gas ○ Increased anteroposterior diameter ○ [Reduced vital capacity] ○ [Tachycardia]

Cardiac Output, decreased

DEFINITION: A state in which the blood pumped by an individual's heart is sufficiently reduced that it is inadequate to meet the needs of the body's tissues.

Note: In a hypermetabolic state, although cardiac output may be within normal range, it may still be inadequate to meet the needs of the body's tissues. Cardiac output and tissue perfusion are interrelated although there are differences. When cardiac output is decreased, tissue perfusion problems will develop; however, tissue perfusion problems can exist without decreased cardiac output.]

■ = critical factors/major signs and symptoms

NOTE: Information appearing in [ ] has been added by the authors to clarify and facilitate the use of nursing diagnoses.

RELATED FACTORS: To be developed by NANDA ○ (Mechanical: alteration in preload [e.g., decreased venous return, altered myocardial contractility]; afterload [e.g., alteration in systemic vascular resistance]; inotropic changes in heart) ○ (Electrical: alterations in rate; rhythm; conduction) ○ (Structural [e.g., ventricular-septal defect, ventricular aneurysm, papillary muscle rupture, valvular disease])

Note: These factors were identified when the diagnosis was originally accepted and have been retained here to assist the user until NANDA completes its work.

DEFINING CHARACTERISTICS

SUBJECTIVE: ○ Fatigue ○ Dyspnea

OBJECTIVE: ○ Variations in blood pressure [and hemodynamic] readings ○ Color changes, skin and mucous membranes [cyanosis] ○ Cold, clammy skin ○ Orthopnea ○ Arrhythmias; [ECG changes] ○ Jugular vein distention ○ Oliguria; anuria ○ Decreased peripheral pulses ○ Rales [crackles] ○ Restlessness

OTHER POSSIBLE CHARACTERISTICS

SUBJECTIVE: ○ Syncope ○ Vertigo ○ Weakness ○ Shortness of breath ○ [Angina]

OBJECTIVE: ○ Edema ○ Change in mental status ○ Frothy sputum ○ Gallop rhythm; abnormal heart sounds ○ Cough ○ [Liver engorgement/ascites]

Caregiver Role Strain

DEFINITION: A caregiver's felt difficulty in performing the family caregiver role.

RELATED FACTORS

PATHOPHYSIOLOGICAL/PHYSIOLOGICAL: ○ Illness severity of the care receiver ○ Addiction or codependency ○ Premature birth/congenital defect ○ Discharge of family member with significant home care needs ○ Caregiver health impairment ○ Unpredictable illness course or instability in the care receiver's health ○ Caregiver is female

DEVELOPMENTAL: ○ Caregiver is not developmentally ready for caregiver role, e.g., young adult needing to provide care for a middle-aged parent ○ Developmental delay or retardation of the care receiver or caregiver

PSYCHOSOCIAL: ○ Psychosocial or cognitive problems in care receiver ○ Marginal family adaptation or dysfunction prior to the caregiving situation ○ Marginal caregiver's coping patterns ○ Past history of poor relationship between caregiver and care receiver ○ Caregiver is spouse ○ Care receiver exhibits deviant, bizarre behavior

SITUATIONAL: ○ Presence of abuse or violence ○ Presence of situational stressors that normally affect families, such as significant loss, disaster or crisis, poverty or economic vulnerability, or major life events, e.g., birth, hospitalization, leaving home, returning home, marriage, divorce, employment, retirement,

---

■ = critical factors/major signs and symptoms

NOTE: Information appearing in [ ] has been added by the authors to clarify and facilitate the use of nursing diagnoses.

death ○ Duration of caregiving required ○ Inadequate physical environment for providing care, e.g., housing, transportation, community services, equipment ○ Family/caregiver isolation ○ Lack of respite and recreation for caregiver ○ Inexperience with caregiving ○ Caregiver's competing role commitments ○ Complexity/amount of caregiving tasks

Note: The presence of this problem may encompass numerous problems/high-risk concerns. Careful attention to data gathering will identify and clarify the client's specific needs, which can then be coordinated under this single diagnostic label.

DEFINING CHARACTERISTICS

SUBJECTIVE: Caregivers report they: ○ Do not have enough resources to provide the care needed ○ Find it hard to do specific caregiving activities ○ Worry about such things as the care receiver's health and emotional state, having to put the care receiver in an institution, and who will care for the care receiver if something should happen to the caregiver ○ Feel [believe] that caregiving interferes with other important roles in their lives such as being a worker, parent, spouse, or friend ○ Feel loss because the care receiver is like a different person compared to before caregiving began or, in the case of a child, that the care receiver was never the child the caregiver expected ○ Feel family conflict around issues of providing care, feeling that other family members do not do their share in providing care to the care receiver, or that not enough appreciation is shown for what the caregiver does ○ Feel stress or nervousness in their relationship with the care receiver ○ Feel depressed

OBJECTIVE: ○ [Inability to meet role expectations/basic needs of caregiver and/or care receiver] ○ [Disorderly surroundings, tasks not done (e.g., bills unpaid)] ○ [Alteration in social participation]

Note: Although objective characteristics were not included in the NANDA diagnosis, if caregiver is in a state of denial, subjective statements may not be made by caregiver; however, statements of care receiver and observations of family members and/or other healthcare providers may indicate presence of problem.

Caregiver Role Strain, risk for*

DEFINITION: A caregiver is vulnerable for felt difficulty in performing the family caregiver role.

RELATED FACTORS

PATHOPHYSIOLOGICAL/PHYSIOLOGICAL: ○ Illness severity of the care receiver ○ Addiction or codependency ○ Premature birth/congenital defect ○ Discharge of family member with significant home care needs ○ Caregiver health impairment

---

■ = critical factors/major signs and symptoms

NOTE: Information appearing in [ ] has been added by the authors to clarify and facilitate the use of nursing diagnoses.

*[**NOTE:** A risk diagnosis is not evidenced by signs and symptoms, since the problem has not yet occurred, and nursing interventions are directed at prevention. Therefore, risk factors present are noted instead.]

○ Unpredictable illness course or instability in the care receiver's health ○ Caregiver is female

DEVELOPMENTAL: ○ Caregiver is not developmentally ready for caregiver role, e.g., young adult needing to provide care for a middle-aged parent ○ Developmental delay or retardation of the care receiver or caregiver

PSYCHOSOCIAL: ○ Psychosocial or cognitive problems in care receiver ○ Marginal family adaptation or dysfunction prior to the caregiving situation ○ Marginal caregiver's coping patterns ○ Past history of poor relationship between caregiver and care receiver ○ Caregiver is spouse ○ Care receiver exhibits deviant, bizarre behavior

SITUATIONAL: ○ Presence of abuse or violence ○ Presence of situational stressors that normally affect families, such as significant loss, disaster or crisis, poverty or economic vulnerability, or major life events, e.g., birth, hospitalization, leaving home, returning home, marriage, divorce, employment, retirement, death ○ Duration of caregiving required ○ Inadequate physical environment for providing care, e.g., housing, transportation, community services, equipment ○ Family/caregiver isolation ○ Lack of respite and recreation for caregiver ○ Inexperience with caregiving ○ Caregiver's competing role commitments ○ Complexity/amount of caregiving tasks

Communication, impaired, verbal

DEFINITION: The state in which an individual experiences a decreased or absent ability to use or understand language in human interaction.

RELATED FACTORS: ○ Decrease in circulation to brain; brain tumor ○ Anatomic deficit, cleft palate ○ Developmental or age-related ○ Physical barrier (tracheostomy, intubation) ○ Psychological barriers (psychosis, lack of stimuli, [depression, panic, anger]) ○ Cultural difference ○ [Drug intake; chemical imbalance]

DEFINING CHARACTERISTICS

SUBJECTIVE: ○ [Reports of difficulty expressing self]

OBJECTIVE: ■ Unable to speak dominant language ■ Speaks or verbalizes with difficulty ■ Does not or cannot speak ○ Disorientation ○ Stuttering; slurring ○ Dyspnea ○ Difficulty forming words or sentences ○ Difficulty expressing thought verbally ○ Inappropriate verbalization, [incessant, loose association of ideas, flight of ideas] ○ [Inability to modulate speech] ○ [Message inappropriate to content] ○ [Use of nonverbal cues, e.g., facial expression, gestures, pleading eyes, turning away] ○ [Frustration, anger, hostility]

Community Coping, enhanced potential for

DEFINITION: A pattern of community activities for adaptation and problem solving that is satisfactory for meeting the demands or needs of the community

---

■ = critical factors/major signs and symptoms

NOTE: Information appearing in [ ] has been added by the authors to clarify and facilitate the use of nursing diagnoses.

but can be improved for management of current and future problems/stressors.

RELATED FACTORS: ○ Social supports available ○ Resources available for problem solving ○ Community has a sense of power to manage stressors

DEFINING CHARACTERISTICS

SUBJECTIVE: ○ Agreement that community is responsible for stress management

OBJECTIVE: ▪ Deficits in one or more characteristics that indicate effective coping ○ Active planning by community for predicted stressors ○ Active problem solving by community when faced with issues ○ Positive communication among community members ○ Positive communication between community/aggregates and larger community ○ Programs available for recreation and relaxation ○ Resources sufficient for managing stressors

Community Coping, ineffective

DEFINITION: A pattern of community activities for adaptation and problem solving that is unsatisfactory for meeting the demands or needs of the community.

RELATED FACTORS: ○ Deficits in social support ○ Inadequate resources for problem solving ○ Powerlessness

DEFINING CHARACTERISTICS

SUBJECTIVE: ○ Community does not meet its own expectations ○ Expressed difficulty in meeting demands for change ○ Expressed vulnerability ○ Stressors perceived as excessive

OBJECTIVE: ○ Deficits of community participation ○ Deficits in communication methods ○ Excessive community conflicts ○ High illness rates

Confusion, acute

DEFINITION: The abrupt onset of a cluster of global, transient changes and disturbances in attention, cognition, psychomotor activity, level of consciousness, and/or sleep/wake cycle.

RELATED FACTORS: ○ Older than 60 years of age ○ Dementia ○ Alcohol abuse ○ Drug abuse ○ Delirium

DEFINING CHARACTERISTICS

OBJECTIVE: ▪ Fluctuation in cognition ▪ Fluctuation in sleep-wake cycle ▪ Fluctuation in level of consciousness ▪ Fluctuation in psychomotor activity ▪ Increased agitation or restlessness ▪ Misperceptions ▪ Lack of motivation to initiate and/or follow through with goal-directed or purposeful behavior ○ Hallucinations

---

▪ = critical factors/major signs and symptoms

NOTE: Information appearing in [ ] has been added by the authors to clarify and facilitate the use of nursing diagnoses.

Confusion, chronic

DEFINITION: An irreversible, long-standing, and/or progressive deterioration of intellect and personality characterized by decreased ability to interpret environmental stimuli, decreased capacity for intellectual thought processes and manifested by disturbances of memory, orientation, and behavior.

RELATED FACTORS: ○ Alzheimer's disease ○ Korsakoff's psychosis ○ Multi-infarct dementia ○ Cerebral vascular accident ○ Head injury

DEFINING CHARACTERISTICS

OBJECTIVE: ■ Clinical evidence of organic impairment ■ Altered interpretation/response to stimuli ■ Progressive/long-standing cognitive impairment ○ No change in level of consciousness ○ Impaired socialization ○ Impaired memory (short term, long term) ○ Altered personality

Constipation

DEFINITION: The state in which an individual experiences a change in normal bowel habits characterized by a decrease in frequency and/or passage of hard, dry stools.

RELATED FACTORS: To be developed by NANDA ○ (Neuromuscular/Musculoskeletal impairment, weak abdominal musculature) ○ (Gastrointestinal obstructive lesions) ○ (Pain on defecation) ○ (Diagnostic procedures) ○ (Pregnancy)

Note: These factors were identified when this diagnosis was originally accepted and have been retained here to assist the user until NANDA completes its work.

DEFINING CHARACTERISTICS

SUBJECTIVE: ○ Frequency less than usual pattern ○ Reported feeling of abdominal or rectal fullness or pressure ○ [Less than usual amount of stool] ○ [Nausea]

OBJECTIVE: ○ Hard-formed stools ○ Straining at stool ○ Palpable mass ○ Decreased activity level, [immobility] ○ [Decreased bowel sounds] ○ [Abdominal distention]

OTHER POSSIBLE CHARACTERISTICS

SUBJECTIVE: ○ Abdominal/back pain ○ Headache ○ Interference with daily living ○ Appetite impairment ○ Use of laxatives ○ [Lack of privacy]

Constipation, colonic

DEFINITION: The state in which an individual's pattern of elimination is characterized by hard, dry stool which results from a delay in passage of food residue.

RELATED FACTORS: ○ Less than adequate fluid/dietary intake; less than adequate fiber ○ Less than adequate physical activity; immobility ○ Lack of privacy;

■ = critical factors/major signs and symptoms

NOTE: Information appearing in [ ] has been added by the authors to clarify and facilitate the use of nursing diagnoses.

change in daily routine ○ Emotional disturbances; stress ○ Chronic use of medication and enemas ○ Metabolic problems, e.g., hypothyroidism, hypocalcemia, hypokalemia

DEFINING CHARACTERISTICS

SUBJECTIVE: ■ Decreased frequency ■ Painful defecation ○ Abdominal pain

OBJECTIVE: ■ Hard, dry stool ■ Straining at stool ■ Abdominal distention ■ Palpable mass ○ Rectal pressure ○ Appetite impairment ○ Headache

Constipation, perceived

DEFINITION: The state in which an individual makes a self-diagnosis of constipation and ensures a daily bowel movement through use of laxatives, enemas, and suppositories.

RELATED FACTORS: ○ Cultural/family health benefits ○ Faulty appraisal ○ Impaired thought processes

DEFINING CHARACTERISTICS

SUBJECTIVE: ■ Expectation of a daily bowel movement with the resulting overuse of laxatives, enemas, and suppositories ■ Expected passage of stool at same time every day

Coping, defensive

DEFINITION: The state in which an individual repeatedly projects falsely positive self-evaluation based on a self-protective pattern which defends against underlying perceived threats to positive self-regard.

RELATED FACTORS: Refer to ND Coping, Individual, ineffective.

DEFINING CHARACTERISTICS

SUBJECTIVE: ■ Denial of obvious problems/weaknesses ■ Projection of blame/responsibility ■ Hypersensitive to slight/criticism ■ Grandiosity ■ Rationalizes failures ○ [Refuses or rejects assistance]

OBJECTIVE: ○ Superior attitude toward others ○ Difficulty establishing/maintaining relationships ○ Hostile laughter or ridicule of others ○ Difficulty in reality testing perceptions ○ Lack of follow-through or participation in treatment or therapy

Coping, Individual, ineffective

DEFINITION: Impairment of adaptive behaviors and problem-solving abilities of a person in meeting life's demands and roles.

RELATED FACTORS: ○ Situational/maturational crises ○ Personal vulnerability ○ Inadequate support systems ○ Poor nutrition ○ Work overload; no vacations; [too

---

■ = critical factors/major signs and symptoms

NOTE: Information appearing in [ ] has been added by the authors to clarify and facilitate the use of nursing diagnoses.

many deadlines] ∘ Unrealistic perceptions ∘ [Multiple stressors, repeated over period of time] ∘ [Multiple life changes; conflict] ∘ [Inadequate relaxation, little or no exercise] ∘ [Unmet expectations] ∘ [Inadequate coping method] ∘ [Impairment of nervous system] ∘ [Memory loss] ∘ [Severe pain, overwhelming threat to self]

DEFINING CHARACTERISTICS

SUBJECTIVE: ▪ Verbalization of inability to cope or inability to ask for help ∘ Reports of chronic worry/anxiety/depression, poor self-esteem ∘ [Reports muscular/emotional tension, lack of appetite, chronic fatigue, insomnia, general irritability]

OBJECTIVE: ▪ Inability to problem-solve ∘ Inability to meet role expectations/basic needs ∘ Alteration in societal participation ∘ Inappropriate use of defense mechanisms ∘ Change in usual communication patterns ∘ Verbal manipulation ∘ High illness rate [including high blood pressure, ulcers, irritable bowel, frequent headaches/neckaches] ∘ High rate of accidents ∘ Destructive behavior toward self or others [including overeating, excessive smoking/drinking, overuse of prescribed medications] ∘ [Lack of assertive behaviors]

Decisional Conflict (specify)

DEFINITION: The state of uncertainty about course of action to be taken when choice among competing actions involves risk, loss, or challenge to personal life values.

RELATED FACTORS: ∘ Unclear personal values/beliefs; perceived threat to value system ∘ Lack of experience or interference with decision-making ∘ Lack of relevant information; multiple or divergent sources of information ∘ Support system deficit

DEFINING CHARACTERISTICS

SUBJECTIVE: Verbalized: ▪ Uncertainty about choices ▪ Undesired consequences of alternative actions being considered ∘ Feelings of distress or questioning personal values and beliefs while attempting a decision

OBJECTIVE: ▪ Vacillation between alternative choices; delayed decision-making ∘ Self-focusing ∘ Physical signs of distress or tension (increased heart rate; increased muscle tension; restlessness etc.)

Denial, ineffective

DEFINITION: The state of a conscious or unconscious attempt to disavow the knowledge or meaning of an event to reduce anxiety/fear to the detriment of health.

RELATED FACTORS: To be developed by NANDA ∘ [Personal vulnerability; unmet self-needs] ∘ [Presence of overwhelming anxiety-producing feelings/situation; reality factors that are consciously intolerable]

▪ = critical factors/major signs and symptoms

NOTE: Information appearing in [ ] has been added by the authors to clarify and facilitate the use of nursing diagnoses.

DEFINING CHARACTERISTICS

SUBJECTIVE: ○ Minimizes symptoms; displaces source of symptoms to other organs ○ Unable to admit impact of disease on life pattern ○ Displaces fear of impact of the condition ○ Does not admit fear of death or invalidism

OBJECTIVE: ▪ Delays seeking or refuses healthcare attention to the detriment of health ▪ Does not perceive personal relevance of symptoms or danger ○ Makes dismissive gestures or comments when speaking of distressing events ○ Displays inappropriate affect ○ Uses home remedies (self-treatment) to relieve symptoms

Diarrhea

DEFINITION: A state in which an individual experiences a change in normal bowel habits characterized by the frequent passage of loose, fluid, unformed stools.

RELATED FACTORS: To be developed by NANDA ○ (Stress and anxiety) ○ (Medications, radiation, toxins, contaminants) ○ (Dietary intake) ○ (Inflammation, irritation, or malabsorption of bowel)

Note: These factors were identified when this diagnosis was originally accepted and have been retained here to assist the user until NANDA completes its work.

DEFINING CHARACTERISTICS

SUBJECTIVE: ○ Abdominal pain ○ Urgency; cramping

OBJECTIVE: ○ Increased frequency ○ Increased frequency of bowel sounds ○ Loose, liquid stools

OTHER POSSIBLE CHARACTERISTICS

OBJECTIVE: ○ Change in color

Disuse Syndrome, risk for*

DEFINITION: A state in which an individual is at risk for deterioration of body systems as the result of prescribed or unavoidable musculoskeletal inactivity.

(**Note:** NANDA-identified complications from immobility can include pressure ulcer, constipation, stasis of pulmonary secretions, thrombosis, urinary tract infection/retention, decreased strength/endurance, orthostatic hypotension, decreased range of joint motion, disorientation, body image disturbance, and powerlessness.)

RISK FACTORS: ○ Severe pain, [chronic pain] ○ Paralysis, [other neuromuscular impairment] ○ Mechanical or prescribed immobilization ○ Altered level of consciousness ○ [Chronic physical or mental illness]

▪ = critical factors/major signs and symptoms

NOTE: Information appearing in [ ] has been added by the authors to clarify and facilitate the use of nursing diagnoses.

*[**NOTE:** A risk diagnosis is not evidenced by signs and symptoms, since the problem has not yet occurred, and nursing interventions are directed at prevention. Therefore, risk factors present are noted instead.]

Diversional Activity deficit

DEFINITION: The state in which an individual experiences a decreased stimulation from or interest or engagement in recreational or leisure activities.

[**Note:** Internal/external factors may or may not be beyond the individual's control.]

RELATED FACTORS: ○ Environmental lack of diversional activity, (e.g., long-term hospitalization; frequent, lengthy treatments, [homebound]) ○ [Physical limitations, bedridden, fatigue, pain] ○ [Situational, developmental problem, lack of resources] ○ [Psychological condition, e.g., depression]

DEFINING CHARACTERISTICS

SUBJECTIVE: Patient's statement regarding the following: ○ Boredom ○ Wish there were something to do, to read, etc. ○ Usual hobbies cannot be undertaken in hospital [or are restricted by physical limitations]

OBJECTIVE: ○ [Flat affect; disinterested] ○ [Restless; crying] [Lethargy; withdrawal] ○ [Hostility] ○ [Overeating or lack of interest in eating] ○ [Weight loss or gain]

Dysreflexia

DEFINITION: The state in which an individual with a spinal cord injury at T7 or above experiences a life-threatening uninhibited sympathetic response of the nervous system to a noxious stimulus.

RELATED FACTORS: ○ Bladder or bowel distention ○ Skin irritation ○ Lack of patient and caregiver knowledge ○ [Sexual excitation]

DEFINING CHARACTERISTICS: ■ Individual with spinal cord injury (T7 or above) with:

SUBJECTIVE: ■ Headache (a diffuse pain in different portions of the head and not confined to any nerve distribution area) ○ Paresthesia ○ Chilling ○ Blurred vision ○ Chest pain ○ Metallic taste in mouth ○ Nasal congestion
OBJECTIVE: ■ Paroxysmal hypertension (sudden periodic elevated BP where systolic pressure is over 140 mm Hg and diastolic is above 90 mm Hg) ■ Bradycardia or tachycardia (pulse rate of less than 60 or over 100 bpm) ■ Diaphoresis (above the injury); red splotches on skin (above the injury); pallor (below the injury) ○ Pilomotor reflex (gooseflesh formation when skin is cooled) ○ Horner's syndrome (contraction of the pupil, partial ptosis of the eyelid, enophthalmos and sometimes loss of sweating over the affected side of the face) ○ Conjunctival congestion

Energy Field disturbance

DEFINITION: A disruption of the flow of energy surrounding a person's being [aura] that results in a disharmony of the body, mind, and/or spirit.

■ = critical factors/major signs and symptoms

NOTE: Information appearing in [ ] has been added by the authors to clarify and facilitate the use of nursing diagnoses.

RELATED FACTORS: [none listed]

DEFINING CHARACTERISISTICS

SUBJECTIVE: ○ Temperature change (warmth/coolness) ○ Visual changes (image/color) ○ Disruption of the field (vacant/hold/spike/bulge) ○ Movement (wave/spike/tingling/dense/flowing) ○ Sounds (tone/words)

Environmental Interpretation Syndrome, impaired

DEFINITION: Consistent lack of orientation to person, place, time, or circumstances over more than 3 to 6 months, necessitating a protective environment.

RELATED FACTORS: ○ Dementia (Alzheimer's disease, Multi-infarct dementia, Pick's disease, AIDS dementia) ○ Parkinson's disease ○ Huntington's disease ○ Depression ○ Alcoholism

DEFINING CHARACTERISTICS

OBJECTIVE: ■ Consistent disorientation in known and unknown environments ■ Chronic confusional states ○ Loss of occupation or social functioning from memory decline ○ Inability to follow simple directions, instructions ○ Inability to reason; concentrate ○ Slow in responding to questions

Family Coping, ineffective: compromised

DEFINITION: A usually supportive primary person (family member or close friend [significant other]) is providing insufficient, ineffective, or compromised support, comfort, assistance, or encouragement which may be needed by the client to manage or master adaptive tasks related to his or her health challenge.

RELATED FACTORS: ○ Inadequate or incorrect information or understanding by a primary person ○ Temporary preoccupation by a significant person who is trying to manage emotional conflicts and personal suffering and is unable to perceive or act effectively in regard to client's needs ○ Temporary family disorganization and role changes ○ Other situation or developmental crises or situations the significant person may be facing ○ Little support provided by client, in turn, for primary person ○ Prolonged disease or disability progression that exhausts the supportive capacity of significant people ○ [Unrealistic expectations of patient/SO of the other] ○ [Lack of mutual decision skills] ○ [Diverse coalitions of family members]

DEFINING CHARACTERISTICS

SUBJECTIVE: ○ Client expresses or confirms a concern or complaint about significant other's response to his or her health problem ○ Significant person describes preoccupation with personal reaction (e.g., fear, anticipatory grief, guilt, anxiety) to client's illness/disability, or to other situation or development crises ○ Significant person describes or confirms an inadequate understanding or knowledge base which interferes with effective assistive or supportive behaviors

---

■ = critical factors/major signs and symptoms

NOTE: Information appearing in [ ] has been added by the authors to clarify and facilitate the use of nursing diagnoses.

OBJECTIVE: ○ Significant person attempts assistive or supportive behaviors with less than satisfactory results ○ Significant person withdraws or enters into limited or temporary personal communication with client at the time of need ○ Significant person displays protective behavior disproportionate (too little or too much) to client's abilities or need for autonomy ○ [Significant person displays sudden outbursts of emotions/shows emotional lability or interferes with necessary nursing/medical interventions]

Family Coping, ineffective: disabling

DEFINITION: Behavior of significant person (family member or other primary person) that disables his or her own capacities and the client's capacities to effectively address tasks essential to either person's adaptation to the health challenge.

RELATED FACTORS: ○ Significant person with chronically unexpressed feelings of guilt, anxiety, hostility, despair, etc. ○ Dissonant discrepancy of coping styles for dealing with adaptive tasks by the significant person and client or among significant people ○ Highly ambivalent family relationships ○ Arbitrary handling of a family's resistance to treatment, which tends to solidify defensiveness as it fails to deal adequately with underlying anxiety

DEFINING CHARACTERISTICS

SUBJECTIVE: ○ [Expresses despair regarding family reactions/lack of involvement]

OBJECTIVE: ○ Intolerance, abandonment, rejection, desertion ○ Psychosomaticism ○ Agitation, depression, aggression, hostility ○ Taking on illness signs of the client ○ Neglectful relationships with other family members ○ Carrying on usual routines disregarding client's needs ○ Neglectful care of the client in regard to basic human needs and/or illness treatment ○ Distortion of reality regarding the client's health problem, including extreme denial about its existence or severity ○ Decisions and actions by family which are detrimental to economic or social well-being ○ Impaired restructuring of a meaningful life for self, impaired individualization, prolonged overconcern for client ○ Client's development of helpless, inactive dependence

Family Coping: potential for growth

DEFINITION: Effective managing of adaptive tasks by family member involved with the client's health challenge, who now is exhibiting desire and readiness for enhanced health and growth in regard to self and in relation to the client.

RELATED FACTORS: ○ Needs sufficiently gratified and adaptive tasks effectively addressed to enable goals of self-actualization to surface ○ [Developmental stage, situational crises/supports]

■ = critical factors/major signs and symptoms

NOTE: Information appearing in [ ] has been added by the authors to clarify and facilitate the use of nursing diagnoses.

DEFINING CHARACTERISTICS

SUBJECTIVE: ◦ Family member attempting to describe growth impact of crisis on his/her own values, priorities, goals, or relationships ◦ Individual expressing interest in making contact on a one-to-one basis or on a mutual-aid group basis with another person who has experienced a similar situation

OBJECTIVE: ◦ Family member moving in direction of health-promoting and enriching lifestyle which supports and monitors maturational processes, audits and negotiates treatment programs, and generally chooses experiences which optimize wellness

Family Process, altered: alcoholism

DEFINITION: The state in which the psychosocial, spiritual, and physiological functions of the family unit are chronically disorganized, leading to conflict, denial of problems, resistance to change, ineffective problem-solving, and a series of self-perpetuating crises.

RELATED FACTORS: ◦ Abuse of alcohol ◦ Family history of alcoholism ◦ Resistance to treatment ◦ Inadequate coping skills ◦ Genetic predisposition ◦ Addictive personality ◦ Lack of problem-solving skills ◦ Biochemical influences

DEFINING CHARACTERISTICS

SUBJECTIVE: Feelings: ■ Decreased self-esteem/worthlessness; ■ Anger/suppressed rage; frustration ■ Powerlessness ■ Anxiety/tension/distress ■ Insecurity ■ Repressed emotions ■ Responsibility for alcoholic's behavior ■ Lingering resentment ■ Shame/embarrassment; guilt ■ Hurt ■ Unhappiness ■ Emotional isolation/loneliness; vulnerability ■ Mistrust ■ Hopelessness ■ Rejection ◦ Being different from other people ◦ Depression ◦ Hostility; fear ◦ Emotional control by others ◦ Confusion ◦ Dissatisfaction ◦ Loss ◦ Misunderstood ◦ Abandonment ◦ Confused love and pity ◦ Moodiness ◦ Failure ◦ Being unloved ◦ Lack of identity

Roles and Relationships: ■ Deterioration in family relationships/disturbed family dynamics ■ Ineffective spouse communication/marital problems ■ Altered role function/disruption of family roles ■ Inconsistent parenting/low perception of parental support ■ Family denial ■ Intimacy dysfunction ■ Chronic family problems ◦ Triangulating family relationships ◦ Reduced ability of family members to relate to each other for mutual growth and maturation ◦ Lack of skills necessary for relationships ◦ Lack of cohesiveness ◦ Disrupted family rituals ◦ Family unable to meet security needs of its members ◦ Pattern of rejection ◦ Economic problems ◦ Neglected obligations

OBJECTIVE: Roles and Relationships: ■ Closed communication systems ◦ Family does not demonstrate respect for individuality and autonomy of its members

Behaviors: ■ Expression of anger inappropriately ■ Difficulty with intimate relationships ■ Loss of control of drinking ■ Alcohol abuse ■ Impaired communication ■ Ineffective problem-solving skills ■ Enabling to maintain drinking

---

■ = critical factors/major signs and symptoms

NOTE: Information appearing in [ ] has been added by the authors to clarify and facilitate the use of nursing diagnoses.

■ Inability to meet emotional needs of its members ■ Manipulation ■ Dependency ■ Criticizing, blaming ■ Broken promises ■ Rationalization/denial of problems ■ Refusal to get help/inability to accept and receive help appropriately ■ Inadequate understanding or knowledge of alcoholism ○ Inability to meet spiritual needs of its members ○ Inability to express or accept wide range of feelings ○ Orientation toward tension relief rather than achievement of goals ○ Family special occasions are centered on alcohol ○ Escalating conflict ○ Lying ○ Contradictory, paradoxical communication ○ Lack of dealing with conflict ○ Harsh self-judgment ○ Isolation ○ Nicotine addiction ○ Difficulty having fun ○ Self-blaming ○ Unresolved grief ○ Controlling communication/power struggles ○ Inability to adapt to change ○ Immaturity ○ Stress-related physical illness ○ Inability to deal with traumatic experiences constructively ○ Seeking approval and affirmation ○ Lack of reliability ○ Disturbances in academic performance in children ○ Disturbances in concentration ○ Chaos ○ Substance abuse other than alcohol ○ Failure to accomplish current or past developmental tasks/difficulty with life cycle transitions ○ Verbal abuse of spouse or parent ○ Agitation ○ Diminished physical contact

Family Processes, altered

DEFINITION: The state in which a family that normally functions effectively experiences a dysfunction.

RELATED FACTORS: ○ Situational transition and/or crises [e.g., economic, change in roles, illness] ○ Developmental transition and/or crises [e.g., loss or gain of a family member]

DEFINING CHARACTERISTICS

SUBJECTIVE: ○ Family uninvolved in community activities ○ Unexamined family myths ○ [Family expresses confusion about what to do, verbalizes they are having difficulty coping with situation]

OBJECTIVE: ○ Family system unable to [does not] meet physical/emotional/spiritual needs of its members ○ Family unable to [does not] meet security needs of its members ○ Inability to accept or receive help appropriately ○ Family unable to [does not] adapt to change or to deal with traumatic experience constructively ○ Parents do not demonstrate respect for each other's views on childrearing practices ○ Inability to express/accept wide range of feelings/feelings of members ○ Inability of family members to relate to each other for mutual growth and maturation ○ Rigidity in function and roles ○ Family does not demonstrate respect for individuality and autonomy of its members ○ Family failing to accomplish current/past development task ○ Unhealthy family decision-making process ○ Failure to send and receive clear messages ○ Inappropriate level and direction of energy ○ Inappropriate boundary maintenance ○ Inappropriate/poorly communicated family rules, rituals, symbols

---

■ = critical factors/major signs and symptoms

NOTE: Information appearing in [ ] has been added by the authors to clarify and facilitate the use of nursing diagnoses.

Fatigue

DEFINITION: An overwhelming sustained sense of exhaustion and decreased capacity for physical and mental work.

RELATED FACTORS: ○ Decreased/increased metabolic energy production ○ Altered body chemistry (e.g., medications; drug withdrawal, chemotherapy) ○ Increased energy requirements to perform activities of daily living ○ Overwhelming psychological or emotional demands ○ Excessive social and/or role demands ○ States of discomfort

DEFINING CHARACTERISTICS

SUBJECTIVE: ■ Verbalization of an unremitting and overwhelming lack of energy; inability to maintain usual routines ○ Perceived need for additional energy to accomplish routine tasks ○ Impaired ability to concentrate ○ Decreased libido

OBJECTIVE: ○ Increase in physical complaints ○ Emotionally labile or irritable ○ Lethargic or listless; disinterest in surroundings/introspection ○ Decreased performance; accident prone

Fear [specify focus]

DEFINITION: Feeling of dread related to an identifiable source which the person validates.

RELATED FACTORS: To be developed by NANDA ○ (Natural or innate origins: environmental stimuli (e.g., sudden noise, loss of physical support, heights, pain) ○ (Learned response: conditioning, modeling from or identification with others) ○ (Separation from support system in a potentially threatening situation such as hospitalization, treatments, etc.) ○ (Knowledge deficit or unfamiliarity) ○ (Phobic stimulus or phobia) ○ (Language barrier [/inability to communicate]) ○ (Sensory impairment) ○ [Threat of death, perceived or actual]
   Note: These factors were identified when this diagnosis was originally accepted and have been retained here to assist the user until NANDA completes its work.

DEFINING CHARACTERISTICS

SUBJECTIVE: ■ Ability to identify object of fear ○ [Panic; scared; jittery] ○ [Increased tension; apprehension; frightened; terrified] ○ [Decreased self-assurance] ○ [Associated physical symptoms; nausea, "heart beating fast," etc.]

OBJECTIVE: ○ [Attack/fight behavior–aggressive; flight behavior–withdrawal] ○ [Impulsiveness] ○ [Wide-eyed; increased alertness; concentration on source] ○ [Sympathetic stimulation: cardiovascular excitation, superficial vasoconstriction, pupil dilation, vomiting, diarrhea, diaphoresis, etc.]

■ = critical factors/major signs and symptoms

NOTE: Information appearing in [ ] has been added by the authors to clarify and facilitate the use of nursing diagnoses.

Fluid Volume deficit [active loss][†]

DEFINITION: The state in which an individual experiences vascular, cellular, or intracellular dehydration [in excess of needs or replacement capabilities due to active loss].

RELATED FACTORS: ○ Active fluid volume loss [e.g., burns, abdominal cancer, hemorrhage, diarrhea, fistulas, use of hyperosmotic radiopaque contrast agents]

DEFINING CHARACTERISTICS

OBJECTIVE: ○ Change in [decreased] urine output ○ Output greater than intake ○ Decreased venous filling ○ Change in [increased] serum sodium ○ Change in [concentrated] urine ○ Sudden weight loss ○ Hemoconcentration

OTHER DEFINING CHARACTERISTICS

SUBJECTIVE: ○ Thirst

OBJECTIVE: ○ Hypotension [postural] ○ Increased pulse rate ○ Decreased skin turgor ○ Decreased pulse volume and pressure ○ Change in mental state ○ Increased body temperature ○ Dry skin/mucous membranes ○ Weakness

Fluid Volume deficit [regulatory failure][†]

DEFINITION: The state in which an individual experiences vascular, cellular, or intracellular dehydration [in excess of needs or replacement capabilities due to failure of regulatory mechanisms].

RELATED FACTORS: ○ Failure of regulator mechanisms [e.g., adrenal disease, recovery phase of acute renal failure, uncontrolled diabetes mellitus/insipidus]

DEFINING CHARACTERISTICS

SUBJECTIVE: ○ [Reports of fatigue, nervousness]

OBJECTIVE: ○ Change in [increased] urine output ○ Change in concentration [dilute] urine ○ Sudden weight loss ○ Decreased venous filling ○ Hemoconcentration ○ Change in serum sodium

OTHER DEFINING CHARACTERISTICS

SUBJECTIVE: ○ Thirst

OBJECTIVE: ○ Hypotension [postural] ○ Increased pulse rate ○ Decreased skin turgor ○ Decreased pulse volume and pressure ○ Change in mental status ○ Increased body temperature ○ Dry skin/mucous membranes ○ Weakness ○ [Edema; possible weight gain]

■ = critical factors/major signs and symptoms

NOTE: Information appearing in [ ] has been added by the authors to clarify and facilitate the use of nursing diagnoses.

[†] **NOTE:** NANDA has combined the originally individual diagnoses of fluid volume deficit, Regulatory Failure and Active Loss. Because the etiology and some interventions for these two diagnoses differ, we have chosen to leave them separate.

Fluid Volume deficit, risk for*

DEFINITION: The state in which an individual is at risk of experiencing vascular, cellular, or intracellular dehydration [due to active or regulatory losses of body water in excess of needs or replacement capability].

RISK FACTORS: ○ Extremes of age and weight ○ Loss of fluid through abnormal routes (e.g., indwelling tubes) ○ Knowledge deficiency related to fluid volume ○ Factors influencing fluid needs (e.g., hypermetabolic states) ○ Medications (e.g., diuretics) ○ Excessive losses through normal routes, (e.g., diarrhea) ○ Deviations affecting access to, intake of, or absorption of fluids (e.g., physical immobility)

Fluid Volume, excess

DEFINITION: The state in which an individual experiences increased fluid retention and edema.

RELATED FACTORS: ○ Compromised regulatory mechanism [e.g., syndrome of inappropriate antidiuretic hormone (SIADH) or decreased plasma proteins (e.g., malnutrition, draining fistulas, burns, organ failure)] ○ Excess fluid intake ○ Excess sodium intake ○ [Drug therapies: e.g., chlorpropamide, tolbutamide, vincristine, triptyline, carbamazepine]

DEFINING CHARACTERISTICS

SUBJECTIVE: ○ Shortness of breath, orthopnea ○ Anxiety

OBJECTIVE: ○ Edema; effusion; anasarca ○ Weight gain ○ Intake greater than output ○ Third (S_3) heart sound ○ Pulmonary congestion (chest x-ray) ○ Abnormal breath sounds, rales (crackles) ○ Change in respiratory pattern ○ Change in mental status; restlessness ○ Blood pressure changes ○ Central venous pressure changes ○ Pulmonary artery pressure changes ○ Jugular venous distention ○ Positive hepatojugular reflex ○ Oliguria; specific gravity changes ○ Azotemia; altered electrolytes ○ Decreased hemoglobin, hematocrit

Gas Exchange, impaired

DEFINITION: The state in which the individual experiences a decreased passage of oxygen and/or carbon dioxide between the alveoli of the lungs and the vascular system. [This may be an entity of its own but may also be an end result of other pathology with an interrelatedness between airway clearance and/or breathing pattern problems.]

RELATED FACTORS: ○ Ventilation perfusion imbalance: ○ [Altered blood flow, e.g., pulmonary embolus, increased vascular resistance] ○ [Alveolar-capillary

---

■ = critical factors/major signs and symptoms

NOTE: Information appearing in [ ] has been added by the authors to clarify and facilitate the use of nursing diagnoses.

*[**NOTE:** A risk diagnosis is not evidenced by signs and symptoms, since the problem has not yet occurred, and nursing interventions are directed at prevention. Therefore, risk factors present are noted instead.]

membrane changes, e.g., adult respiratory distress syndrome; chronic conditions, such as pneumonoconiosis, asbestosis/silicosis] ○ [Altered oxygen supply, e.g., altitude sickness] ○ [Altered oxygen-carrying capacity of blood, e.g., Sickle cell/other anemia, carbon monoxide poisoning]

DEFINING CHARACTERISTICS

SUBJECTIVE: ○ [Dyspnea] ○ [Sense of impending doom]

OBJECTIVE: ○ Confusion ○ Restlessness ○ Inability to move secretions ○ Hypoxia ○ Somnolence ○ Irritability ○ Hypercapnea ○ [Cyanosis] ○ [Tachycardia] ○ [Polycythemia]

Grieving, anticipatory

DEFINITION: [Response to loss before it actually occurs. **Note:** May be a healthy response requiring interventions of support and information-giving.]

RELATED FACTORS: To be developed by NANDA ○ [Perceived potential loss of: significant other, physiopsychosocial well-being, personal possessions]

DEFINING CHARACTERISTICS

SUBJECTIVE: ○ Sorrow; guilt; anger; choked feelings ○ Denial of potential loss ○ Expression of distress at potential loss ○ Alterations in activity level; sleep patterns ○ Changes in eating habits ○ Altered libido

OBJECTIVE: ○ Potential loss of significant object ○ Altered communication patterns ○ [Altered affect] ○ [Crying] ○ [Social isolation, altered activity levels, withdrawal]

Grieving, dysfunctional

DEFINITION: [Delayed or exaggerated response to a perceived, actual, or potential loss.]

RELATED FACTORS: ○ Actual or perceived object loss (object loss is used in the broadest sense) and may include people, possessions, a job, status, home, ideals, parts and processes of the body [e.g., amputation, paralysis, chronic/ fatal illness] ○ [Thwarted grieving response to a loss] ○ [Lack of resolution of previous grieving response] ○ [Absence of anticipatory grieving]

DEFINING CHARACTERISTICS

SUBJECTIVE: ○ Verbal expression of distress at loss ○ Expression of unresolved issues ○ Idealization of lost object ○ Denial of loss ○ Anger; sadness ○ Alterations in: eating habits, sleep and dream patterns, activity levels, libido ○ Reliving of past experiences ○ Expression of guilt ○ [Hopelessness]

OBJECTIVE: ○ Crying ○ Difficulty in expressing loss ○ Interference with life functioning ○ Alterations in concentration and/or pursuits of tasks ○ Labile affect ○ Developmental regression ○ [Isolation]

■ = critical factors/major signs and symptoms

NOTE: Information appearing in [ ] has been added by the authors to clarify and facilitate the use of nursing diagnoses.

Growth and Development, altered

DEFINITION: The state in which an individual demonstrates deviations in norms from his/her age group.

RELATED FACTORS: ○ Inadequate caretaking [physical/emotional neglect/abuse] ○ Indifference, inconsistent responsiveness, multiple caretakers ○ Separation from significant other(s) ○ Environmental and stimulation deficiencies ○ Effects of physical disability [handicapping condition] ○ Prescribed dependence ○ [Insufficient expectations for self-care] ○ [Prolonged/painful treatments; prolonged/repeated hospitalizations] ○ [Physical/emotional illness (chronic, traumatic)]

DEFINING CHARACTERISTICS

SUBJECTIVE: ■ Inability to perform self-care or self-control activities appropriate for age [■ Regression/loss of previously acquired skills; precocious or accelerated skill attainment]

OBJECTIVE: ■ Delay or difficulty in performing skills (motor, social, or expressive) typical of age group ■ Altered physical growth ○ Flat affect ○ Listlessness, decreased responses ○ [Sleep disturbances, negative mood/responses]

Health Maintenance, altered

DEFINITION: Inability to identify, manage, and/or seek out help to maintain health. [This diagnosis contains components of other nursing diagnoses. We recommend subsuming health maintenance interventions under the "basic" nursing diagnosis when a single causative factor is identified, e.g., Knowledge deficit [Learning Need] (specify); Communication, impaired: verbal; Thought processes, altered; Individual/Family Coping, ineffective.]

RELATED FACTORS: ○ Lack of or significant alteration in communication skills (written, verbal, and/or gestural) ○ Unachieved development tasks ○ Lack of ability to make deliberate and thoughtful judgments ○ Perceptual or cognitive impairment ○ Complete or partial lack of gross and/or fine motor skills) ○ Ineffective individual/family coping ○ Dysfunctional grieving; disabling spiritual distress ○ Lack of material resource

DEFINING CHARACTERISTICS

SUBJECTIVE: ○ Expressed interest in improving health behaviors ○ Reported or observed lack of equipment, financial, and/or other resources ○ Reported or observed impairment of personal support system ○ [Reported or observed compulsive behaviors]

OBJECTIVE: ○ Demonstrated lack of knowledge regarding basic health practices ○ Reported or observed inability to take the responsibility for meeting basic health practices in any or all functional pattern areas ○ Demonstrated lack of adaptive behaviors to internal/external environmental changes ○ History of lack of health-seeking behavior

---

■ = critical factors/major signs and symptoms

NOTE: Information appearing in [ ] has been added by the authors to clarify and facilitate the use of nursing diagnoses.

Health Seeking Behaviors [specify]

DEFINITION: A state in which an individual in stable health is actively seeking ways to alter personal health habits and/or the environment in order to move toward higher level of health. (Stable health status is defined as age appropriate illness prevention measures achieved, client reports good or excellent health, and signs and symptoms of disease if present are controlled.)

RELATED FACTORS: ○ [Situational/maturational occurrence precipitating concern about current health status]

DEFINING CHARACTERISTICS

SUBJECTIVE: ■ Expressed desire to seek a higher level of wellness ○ Expressed desire to modify codependent behaviors ○ Expressed desire for increased control of health practice ○ Expression of concern about current environmental conditions on health status ○ Stated (or observed) unfamiliarity with wellness community resources

OBJECTIVE: ■ Observed desire to seek a higher level of wellness ○ Observed desire for increased control of health practice ○ Demonstrated or observed lack of knowledge in health promotion behaviors

Home Maintenance Management, impaired

DEFINITION: Inability to independently maintain a safe, growth-promoting immediate environment.

RELATED FACTORS: ○ Individual/family member disease or injury ○ Insufficient family organization or planning ○ Insufficient finances ○ Impaired cognitive or emotional functioning ○ Lack of role modeling ○ Unfamiliarity with neighborhood resources ○ Lack of knowledge ○ Inadequate support systems

DEFINING CHARACTERISTICS

SUBJECTIVE: Household members: ■ Express difficulty in maintaining their home in a comfortable fashion ■ Request assistance with home maintenance ■ Describe outstanding debts or financial crises

OBJECTIVE: ■ Accumulation of dirt, food, or hygienic wastes ■ Unwashed or unavailable cooking equipment, clothes, or linen ■ Overtaxed family members (e.g., exhausted, anxious) ■ Repeated hygienic disorders, infestations, or infections ○ Disorderly surroundings ○ Inappropriate household temperature ○ Lack of necessary equipment or aids ○ Presence of vermin or rodents ○ Offensive odors

Hopelessness

DEFINITION: A subjective state in which an individual sees limited or no alternatives or personal choices available and is unable to mobilize energy on own behalf.

■ = critical factors/major signs and symptoms

NOTE: Information appearing in [ ] has been added by the authors to clarify and facilitate the use of nursing diagnoses.

RELATED FACTORS: ○ Prolonged activity restriction creating isolation ○ Failing or deteriorating physiologic condition ○ Long-term stress; abandonment ○ Lost belief in transcendent values/God

DEFINING CHARACTERISTICS

SUBJECTIVE: ▪ Verbal cues (despondent content, "I can't," sighing)

OBJECTIVE: ▪ Passivity, decreased verbalization ▪ Decreased affect ○ Lack of initiative ○ Decreased response to stimuli ○ Turning away from speaker ○ Closing eyes ○ Shrugging in response to speaker ○ Decreased appetite, increased/decreased sleep ○ Lack of involvement in care/passively allowing care [▪ Withdrawal from environs] ○ [Lack of involvement/interest in significant other(s) (children, spouse)] ○ [Angry outbursts]

Hyperthermia

DEFINITION: A state in which an individual's body temperature is elevated above his/her normal range.

RELATED FACTORS: ○ Exposure to hot environment; inappropriate clothing ○ Vigorous activity; dehydration ○ Inability or decreased ability to perspire ○ Medications/anesthesia ○ Increased metabolic rate; illness or trauma

DEFINING CHARACTERISTICS

SUBJECTIVE: ○ [Headache]

OBJECTIVE: ▪ Increase in body temperature above normal range ○ Flushed skin, warm to touch ○ Increased respiratory rate, tachycardia ○ Seizures/convulsions ○ [Unstable blood pressure] ○ [Muscle rigidity/fasciculations] ○ [Confusion]

Hypothermia

DEFINITION: The state in which an individual's body temperature is reduced below normal range.

RELATED FACTORS: ○ Exposure to cool or cold environment, [prolonged exposure, immersion in cold water/near drowning, artificial hypothermia/cardiopulmonary bypass] ○ Inadequate clothing ○ Evaporation from skin in cool environment ○ Inability or decreased ability to shiver ○ Aging [or very young] ○ [Debilitating] illness or trauma, damage to hypothalamus ○ Malnutrition; decreased metabolic rate; inactivity ○ Consumption of alcohol; medications causing vasodilation ○ [Vasodilation, e.g., sepsis, drug overdose]

DEFINING CHARACTERISTICS

SUBJECTIVE ▪ Reduction in body temperature below normal range ▪ Shivering (mild) ▪ Cool skin ▪ Pallor (moderate) ○ Slow capillary refill ○ Cyanotic nail beds ○ Hypertension; tachycardia ○ Piloerection ○ [Core temperature 95°F: de-

---

▪ = critical factors/major signs and symptoms

NOTE: Information appearing in [ ] has been added by the authors to clarify and facilitate the use of nursing diagnoses.

creased pulse, increased respiration, poor judgment, memory loss] ○ [Core temperature 94° to 90.5°F: all vital signs decreased, myocardial irritability/dysrhythmias, muscle rigidity, no shivering, obtunded] ○ [Core temperature 85°F: no apparent vital signs, heart rate unresponsive to drug therapy, cyanotic, dilated pupils, appears dead]

Incontinence, functional

DEFINITION: The state in which an individual experiences an involuntary, unpredictable passage of urine.

RELATED FACTORS: ○ Altered environment [e.g., poor lighting or inability to locate bathroom] ○ Sensory, cognitive [e.g., inattentiveness to urge to void, use of sedation], or mobility deficits [including difficulty in removing clothes] ○ [Increased urine production] ○ [Reluctance to use call light or bedpan]

DEFINING CHARACTERISTICS

SUBJECTIVE: ■ Urge to void or bladder contractions sufficiently strong to result in loss of urine before reaching an appropriate receptacle ○ [Voiding in large amounts]

Incontinence, reflex

DEFINITION: The state in which an individual experiences an involuntary loss of urine, occurring at somewhat predictable intervals when a specific bladder volume is reached.

RELATED FACTORS: ○ Neurologic impairment (e.g., spinal cord lesion which interferes with conduction of cerebral messages above the level of the reflex arc) ○ [Cerebral lesion abolishing voluntary control]

DEFINING CHARACTERISTICS

SUBJECTIVE: ■ No [or only partial] awareness of bladder filling ■ No urge to void or feelings of bladder fullness ○ [Voids in large amounts] ○ [Unaware of being incontinent]

OBJECTIVE: ■ Uninhibited bladder contraction/spasm at regular intervals

Incontinence, stress

DEFINITION: The state in which an individual experiences a loss of urine of less than 50 mL occurring with increased abdominal pressure.

RELATED FACTORS: ○ Degenerative changes in pelvic muscles and structural supports associated with increased age ○ High intra-abdominal pressure (e.g., obesity, gravid uterus) ○ Incompetent bladder outlet ○ Overdistention between voidings ○ Weak pelvic muscles and structural supports

---

■ = critical factors/major signs and symptoms

NOTE: Information appearing in [ ] has been added by the authors to clarify and facilitate the use of nursing diagnoses.

DEFINING CHARACTERISTICS

SUBJECTIVE: ▪ Reported dribbling with increased abdominal pressure [e.g., coughing, sneezing, lifting, impact aerobics, changing position] ○ Urinary urgency/frequency (more often than every 2 hours)

OBJECTIVE: ▪ Observed dribbling with increased abdominal pressure

Incontinence, total

DEFINITION: The state in which an individual experiences a continuous and unpredictable loss of urine.

RELATED FACTORS: ○ Neuropathy preventing transmission of reflex [signals to the reflex arc] indicating bladder fullness ○ Neurologic dysfunction causing triggering of micturition at unpredictable times [cerebral lesions] ○ Independent contraction of detrusor reflex due to surgery ○ Trauma or disease affecting spinal cord nerves [destruction of sensory or motor neurons below the injury level] ○ Anatomic (fistula)

DEFINING CHARACTERISTICS

SUBJECTIVE: ▪ Constant flow of urine occurs at unpredictable times without distention or uninhibited bladder contractions/spasm ▪ Nocturia ○ Lack of perineal or bladder filling awareness ○ Unawareness of incontinence

OBJECTIVE: ▪ Unsuccessful incontinence refractory treatments

Incontinence, urge

DEFINITION: The state in which an individual experiences involuntary passage of urine occurring soon after a strong sense of urgency to void.

RELATED FACTORS: ○ Decreased bladder capacity (e.g., history of PID, abdominal surgeries, indwelling urinary catheter) ○ Irritation of bladder stretch receptors causing spasm (e.g., bladder infection); alcohol; caffeine; increased fluids; increased urine concentration; overdistention of bladder

DEFINING CHARACTERISTICS

SUBJECTIVE: ▪ Urinary urgency ▪ Frequency (voiding more often than every 2 hours) ▪ Bladder contracture/spasm ○ Nocturia (more than two times per night)

OBJECTIVE: ▪ Inability to reach toilet in time ○ Voiding in small amounts (less than 100 mL) or in large amounts (more than 550 mL)

Infant Behavior, disorganized

DEFINITION: Alteration in integration and modulation of the physiological and behavioral systems of functioning (i.e., autonomic, motor, state, organizational, self-regulatory, and attentional-interactional systems).

▪ = critical factors/major signs and symptoms

NOTE: Information appearing in [ ] has been added by the authors to clarify and facilitate the use of nursing diagnoses.

RELATED FACTORS: ○ Pain ○ Oral/motor problems ○ Feeding intolerance ○ Environmental overstimulation ○ Lack of containment/boundaries ○ Prematurity ○ Invasive/painful procedures

DEFINING CHARACTERISTICS

OBJECTIVE: ■ Change from baseline physiological measures ■ Tremors, startles, twitches ■ Hyperextension of arms and legs ■ Diffuse/unclear sleep ■ Deficient self-regulatory behaviors ■ Deficient response to visual/auditory stimuli ○ Yawning ○ Apnea

Infant Behavior, disorganized, risk for*

DEFINITION: Risk for alteration in integration and modulation of the physiological and behavioral systems of functioning (i.e., autonomic, motor, state, organizational, self-regulatory, and attentional-interactional systems).

RISK FACTORS: ○ Pain ○ Oral/motor problems ○ Environmental overstimulation ○ Lack of containment/boundaries ○ Prematurity ○ Invasive/painful procedures

Infant Behavior, organized, potential for enhancement

DEFINITION: A pattern of modulation of the physiological and behavioral systems of functioning of an infant (i.e., autonomic, motor, state, organizational, self-regulatory, and attentional-interactional systems) that is satisfactory but can be improved, resulting in higher levels of integration in response to environmental stimuli.

RELATED FACTORS: ○ Prematurity ○ Pain

DEFINING CHARACTERISTICS

OBJECTIVE: ○ Stable physiological measures ○ Definite sleep-wake states ■ Use of some self-regulatory behaviors ○ Response to visual/auditory stimuli

Infant Feeding Pattern, ineffective

DEFINITION: A state in which an infant demonstrates an impaired ability to suck or coordinate the suck-swallow response

RELATED FACTORS: ○ Prematurity ○ Neurologic impairment/delay ○ Oral hypersensitivity ○ Prolonged NPO ○ Anatomic abnormality

DEFINING CHARACTERISTICS

SUBJECTIVE: ○ [Mother reports infant is unable to initiate or sustain an effective suck]

OBJECTIVE: ■ Inability to initiate or sustain an effective suck ■ Inability to coordinate sucking, swallowing, and breathing

---

■ = critical factors/major signs and symptoms

NOTE: Information appearing in [ ] has been added by the authors to clarify and facilitate the use of nursing diagnoses.

*[**NOTE:** A risk diagnosis is not evidenced by signs and symptoms, since the problem has not yet occurred, and nursing interventions are directed at prevention. Therefore, risk factors present are noted instead.]

Infection, risk for*

DEFINITION: The state in which an individual is at increased risk for being invaded by pathogenic organisms.

RISK FACTORS: ○ Inadequate primary defenses (broken skin, traumatized tissue, decrease in ciliary action, stasis of body fluids, change in pH secretions, altered peristalsis) ○ Inadequate secondary defenses (e.g., decreased hemoglobin, leukopenia, suppressed inflammatory response) and immunosuppression ○ Inadequate acquired immunity; tissue destruction and increased environmental exposure ○ Chronic disease; malnutrition; trauma ○ Invasive procedures ○ Pharmaceutical agents [including antibiotic therapy] ○ Rupture of amniotic membranes ○ Insufficient knowledge to avoid exposure to pathogens

Injury, risk for*

DEFINITION: A state in which the individual is at risk of injury as a result of environmental conditions interacting with the individual's adaptive and defensive resources. [**Note:** The potential for injury differs from individual to individual and situation to situation. It is our belief that the environment is not safe, and there is no way to list everything that might present a danger to someone. Rather, we believe nurses have the responsibility to educate people throughout their life cycles to live safely in their environment.]

RISK FACTORS

INTERNAL: ○ Biochemical, regulatory function: (sensory, integrative, effector dysfunction; tissue hypoxia); malnutrition; immune-autoimmune; abnormal blood profile, (leukocytosis/leukopenia; altered clotting factors, thrombocytopenia; sickle cell, thalassemia; decreased hemoglobin) ○ Physical: (broken skin, altered mobility); developmental age; (physiologic, psychosocial) ○ Psychological: (affective, orientation)

EXTERNAL: ○ Biological (immunization level of community, microorganism) ○ Chemical: (pollutants, poisons, drugs, pharmaceutical agents, alcohol, caffeine, nicotine, preservatives, cosmetics and dyes), nutrients (vitamins, food types) ○ Physical: (design, structure, and arrangement of community, building, and/or equipment); mode of transport/transportation ○ People-provider: (nosocomial agent, staffing patterns; cognitive, affective, and psychomotor factors)

Knowledge deficit [Learning Need] (specify)

DEFINITION: [Lack of specific information necessary for patient/SO to make informed choices regarding condition/therapies/treatment plan]

RELATED FACTORS: ○ Lack of exposure ○ Information misinterpretation ○ Unfamiliarity with information resources ○ Lack of recall ○ Cognitive limitation ○ Lack

---

■ = critical factors/major signs and symptoms

NOTE: Information appearing in [ ] has been added by the authors to clarify and facilitate the use of nursing diagnoses.

*[**NOTE:** A risk diagnosis is not evidenced by signs and symptoms, since the problem has not yet occurred, and nursing interventions are directed at prevention. Therefore, risk factors present are noted instead.]

of interest in learning ○ [Patient's request for no information] ○ [Inaccurate/ incomplete information presented]

DEFINING CHARACTERISTICS

SUBJECTIVE: ○ Verbalization of the problem ○ [Request for information] ○ [Statement of misconception]

OBJECTIVE: ○ Inaccurate follow-through of instruction ○ Inadequate performance of test ○ Inappropriate or exaggerated behaviors (e.g., hysterical, hostile, agitated, apathetic) ○ [Development of preventable complication]

Loneliness, risk for*

DEFINITION: A subjective state in which an individual is at risk of experiencing vague dysphoria.

RISK FACTORS: ○ Affectional deprivation ○ Physical isolation ○ Cathectic deprivation ○ Social isolation

Memory, impaired

DEFINITION: The state in which an individual experiences the inability to remember or recall bits of information or behavioral skills. Impaired memory may be attributed to physiopathological or situational causes that are either temporary or permanent.

RELATED FACTORS: ○ Acute or chronic hypoxia ○ Anemia ○ Decreased cardiac output ○ Fluid and electrolyte imbalance ○ Neurological disturbances ○ Excessive environmental disturbances

DEFINING CHARACTERISTICS

SUBJECTIVE: ■ Reported experiences of forgetting ■ Inability to recall recent or past events

OBJECTIVE: ■ Observed experiences of forgetting ■ Inability to determine if a behavior was performed ■ Inability to learn or retain new skills or information ■ Inability to perform a previously learned skill ■ Inability to perform a previously learned skill ■ Inability to recall factual information

Noncompliance [Compliance, altered] (specify)

DEFINITION: A person's informed decision not to adhere to a therapeutic recommendation. [**Note:** Noncompliance is a term that may create a negative situation for patient and caregiver that may foster difficulties in resolving the

---

■ = critical factors/major signs and symptoms

NOTE: Information appearing in [ ] has been added by the authors to clarify and facilitate the use of nursing diagnoses.

*[**NOTE:** A risk diagnosis is not evidenced by signs and symptoms, since the problem has not yet occurred, and nursing interventions are directed at prevention. Therefore, risk factors present are noted instead.]

causative factors. Since patients have a right to refuse therapy, we see this as a situation in which the professional need is to accept the patient's point of view/behavior/choice(s) and work together to find alternate means to meet original and/or revised goals.]

RELATED FACTORS: ○ Patient value system: health beliefs, cultural influences, spiritual values ○ Client-provider relationships ○ [Fear/Anxiety] ○ [Altered thought processes, e.g., depression, paranoia] ○ [Difficulty changing behavior, e.g., addictions] ○ [Inadequate resources, support systems]

DEFINING CHARACTERISTICS

SUBJECTIVE: ■ Statements by patient or significant other(s), [e.g., does not perceive illness/risk to be serious, does not believe in efficacy of therapy; unwillingness to follow treatment regimen or accept side effects, restrictions] ○ [Denial]

OBJECTIVE: ■ Behavior indicative of failure to adhere (by direct observation) ○ Objective tests (physiologic measures, detection of markers) ○ Failure to progress ○ Evidence of development of complications; exacerbation of symptoms ○ Failure to keep appointments ○ [Inability to set or attain mutual goals]

Nutrition, altered, less than body requirements

DEFINITION: The state in which an individual experiences an intake of nutrients insufficient to meet metabolic needs.

RELATED FACTORS: ○ Inability to ingest or digest food or absorb nutrients due to biological, psychological, or economic factors ○ [Lack of information regarding individual needs] ○ [Intake insufficient to meet increased metabolic demands]

DEFINING CHARACTERISTICS

SUBJECTIVE: ○ Reported inadequate food intake less than RDA ○ Reported or evidence of lack of food ○ Lack of interest in food ○ Aversion to eating ○ Reported altered taste sensation ○ Perceived inability to ingest food ○ Satiety immediately after ingesting food ○ Abdominal cramping ○ Abdominal pain with or without pathology ○ Lack of information, misinformation, misconceptions [authors view this as a Related Factor]

OBJECTIVE: ○ Body weight 20 percent or more under ideal [for height and frame] ○ Loss of weight with adequate food intake ○ Poor muscle tone ○ Weakness of muscles required for swallowing or mastication ○ Sore, inflamed buccal cavity ○ Capillary fragility ○ Hyperactive bowel sounds ○ Diarrhea and/or steatorrhea ○ Pale conjunctiva and mucous membranes ○ Excessive loss of hair [or increased growth of hair on body (lanugo)] ○ [Decreased subcutaneous fat/muscle mass] ○ [Cessation of menses]

Nutrition, altered, more than body requirements

DEFINITION: The state in which an individual is experiencing an intake of nutrients which exceeds metabolic needs.

■ = critical factors/major signs and symptoms

NOTE: Information appearing in [ ] has been added by the authors to clarify and facilitate the use of nursing diagnoses.

RELATED FACTORS: ○ Excessive intake in relationship to metabolic need [**Note:** Underlying cause is often complex and may be difficult to diagnose/treat]

DEFINING CHARACTERISTICS

SUBJECTIVE: ○ Reported dysfunctional eating patterns:

Pairing food with other activities
Eating in response to external cues such as time of day, social situation
Concentrating food intake at end of day
Eating in response to internal cues other than hunger, for example, anxiety

○ Sedentary activity level

OBJECTIVE: ○ Weight 10 percent over ideal for height and frame [overweight] ■ Weight 20 percent over ideal for height and frame [obese] ■ Triceps skin fold greater than 15 mm in men and 25 mm in women ○ Observed dysfunctional eating patterns [as noted in Subjective] ○ [Percentage of body fat greater than: 18 to 20 percent for trim women; 10 to 12 percent for trim men.]

Nutrition, altered, risk for more than body requirements*

DEFINITION: The state in which an individual is at risk of experiencing an intake of nutrients which exceeds metabolic needs.

RISK FACTORS: ■ Reported/observed obesity in one or both parents [/spouse; hereditary predisposition] ■ Rapid transition across growth percentiles in infants or children, [adolescence] ○ Reported use of solid food as major food source before 5 months of age ○ Reported/observed higher base-line weight at beginning of each pregnancy ○ Dysfunctional eating patterns:

Pairing food with other activities;
Eating in response to external cues such as time of day or social situation;
Concentrating food intake at end of day;
Eating in response to internal cues other than hunger, for example, anxiety

○ Observed use of food as reward or comfort measure ○ [Socially/culturally isolated; lacking other outlets] ○ [Alteration in usual activity patterns/sedentary lifestyle] ○ [Alteration in usual coping patterns] ○ [Majority of foods consumed are concentrated, high-calorie or fat sources] ○ [Significant/sudden decline in financial resources, lower socioeconomic status]

Oral Mucous Membrane, altered

DEFINITION: The state in which the individual experiences disruptions in the tissue layers of the oral cavity.

■ = critical factors/major signs and symptoms

NOTE: Information appearing in [ ] has been added by the authors to clarify and facilitate the use of nursing diagnoses.

*[**NOTE:** A risk diagnosis is not evidenced by signs and symptoms, since the problem has not yet occurred, and nursing interventions are directed at prevention. Therefore, risk factors present are noted instead.]

RELATED FACTORS: ○ Pathological conditions: oral cavity (radiation to head and/or neck) ○ Trauma (chemical, e.g., acidic foods, drugs, noxious agents, alcohol; mechanical, e.g., ill-fitting dentures, braces, tubes (endotracheal, nasogastric), surgery (in oral cavity) ○ NPO for more than 24 hours ○ Lack of or decreased salivation ○ Mouth breathing ○ Ineffective oral hygiene; infection ○ Medication ○ Malnutrition ○ Dehydration

DEFINING CHARACTERISTICS

SUBJECTIVE: ○ Xerostomia (dry mouth) ○ Oral pain/discomfort

OBJECTIVE: ○ Lack of or decreased salivation ○ Coated tongue ○ Stomatitis; leukoplakia; hyperemia ○ Hemorrhagic gingivitis; vesicles ○ Halitosis ○ Carious teeth ○ Oral plaque lesions or ulcers; desquamation ○ Edema

Pain [acute]

DEFINITION: A state in which an individual experiences and reports the presence of severe discomfort or an uncomfortable sensation.

RELATED FACTORS: ○ Injuring agents (biologic, chemical, physical, psychological)

DEFINING CHARACTERISTICS

SUBJECTIVE: ○ Communication (verbal or coded) of pain descriptors [expect less from under age 40, males, and some cultural groups] ○ [Pain unrelieved and/or increased beyond tolerance]

OBJECTIVE: ○ Distraction behavior (moaning, crying, pacing, seeking out other people and/or activities, restlessness) ○ Guarding behavior, protective ○ Alteration in muscle tone (may span from listless to rigid) ○ Facial mask of pain (eyes lack luster, "beaten look," fixed or scattered movement, grimace) ○ Autonomic responses not seen in chronic, stable pain (diaphoresis, blood pressure and pulse change, pupillary dilation, increased or decreased respiratory rate) ○ Self-focusing ○ Narrowed focus (altered time perception, withdrawal from social contact, impaired thought process) ○ [Fear/panic]

Pain, chronic

DEFINITION: A state in which the individual experiences pain that continues for more than 6 months in duration. [Pain is a signal that something is wrong. Chronic pain can be recurrent and periodically disabling (e.g., migraine headaches), or may be unremitting. While chronic pain syndrome includes various learned behaviors, psychological factors become the primary contribution to impairment. It is a complex, separate entity, combining elements from other NDs: Powerlessness; Diversional Activity, altered; Family Processes, altered, Self Care deficit (specify): feeding, bathing/hygiene, dressing/grooming, toileting]

RELATED FACTORS: ○ Chronic physical/psychosocial disability

■ = critical factors/major signs and symptoms

NOTE: Information appearing in [ ] has been added by the authors to clarify and facilitate the use of nursing diagnoses.

DEFINING CHARACTERISTICS

SUBJECTIVE: ▪ Verbal report of pain experienced for more than 6 months ○ Fear of reinjury ○ Altered ability to continue previous activities ○ Anorexia, weight changes ○ Changes in sleep patterns ○ [Preoccupation with pain] ○ [Desperately seeks alternative solutions/therapies for relief/control of pain]

OBJECTIVE: ▪ Observed evidence of pain experienced for more than 6 months ○ Physical and social withdrawal ○ Facial mask, guarded movement

Parent/Infant/Child Attachment, altered, risk for*

DEFINITION: Disruption of the interactive process between parent/significant other and infant that fosters the development of a protective and nurturing reciprocal relationship.

RISK FACTORS: ○ Inability of parents to meet the personal needs ○ Anxiety associated with the parent role ○ Substance abuse ○ Premature infant ○ Ill infant/child who is unable to effectively initiate parental contact due to altered behavioral organization ○ Separation ○ Physical barriers ○ Lack of privacy

Parental Role Conflict

DEFINITION: The state in which a parent experiences role confusion and conflict in response to crisis.

RELATED FACTORS: ○ Separation from child due to chronic illness ○ Intimidation with invasive or restrictive modalities (e.g., isolation, intubation) specialized care centers, policies ○ Home care of a child with special needs (e.g., apnea monitoring, postural drainage, hyperalimentation) ○ Change in marital status ○ Interruptions of family life due to home care regimen (treatments, caregivers, lack of respite)

DEFINING CHARACTERISTICS

SUBJECTIVE: Parent(s): ▪ Expresses concerns/feelings of inadequacy to provide for child's physical and emotional needs during hospitalization or in the home ▪ Express concerns about changes in parental role, family functioning, family communication, family health ○ Express concern about perceived loss of control over decisions relating to their child ○ Verbalize feelings of guilt, anger, fear, anxiety, and/or frustrations about effect of child's illness on family process

OBJECTIVE: ▪ Demonstrated disruption in caretaking routines ○ Reluctant to participate in usual care taking activities even with encouragement and support ○ Demonstrate feelings of guilt, anger, fear, anxiety, and/or frustrations about effect of child's illness on family process

---

▪ = critical factors/major signs and symptoms

NOTE: Information appearing in [ ] has been added by the authors to clarify and facilitate the use of nursing diagnoses.

*[**NOTE:** A risk diagnosis is not evidenced by signs and symptoms, since the problem has not yet occurred, and nursing interventions are directed at prevention. Therefore, risk factors present are noted instead.]

Parenting, altered

DEFINITION: The state in which a nurturing figure(s) experiences an inability to create an environment which promotes the optimum growth and development of another human being. (It is important to state as a preface to this diagnosis that adjustment to parenting in general is a normal maturational process that elicits nursing behaviors of prevention of potential problems and health promotion.)

RELATED FACTORS: ○ Lack of available role model; ineffective role model ○ Lack of support between/from significant other(s) ○ Interruption in bonding process, (i.e., maternal, paternal, other) ○ Mental and/or physical illness ○ Lack of knowledge ○ Limited cognitive functioning ○ Multiple pregnancies ○ Unrealistic expectation for self, infant, partner ○ Physical and psychosocial abuse of nurturing figure ○ Unmet social/emotional maturation needs of parenting figures ○ Perceived threat to own survival, physical and emotional ○ Presence of stress (financial, legal, recent crisis, cultural move [e.g., from another country, nationality]) ○ Lack of role identity ○ Lack of appropriate response of child to relationship

DEFINING CHARACTERISTICS

SUBJECTIVE: ■ Verbalization cannot control child ○ Constant verbalization of disappointment in gender or physical characteristics of the infant/child ○ Verbalization of resentment toward the infant/child ○ Verbalization of role inadequacy [inability to care for/discipline child] ○ Verbal disgust at body functions of infant/child ○ Verbalizes desire to have child call him/herself by first name versus traditional cultural tendencies

OBJECTIVE: ■ Incidence of physical and psychologic trauma ■ Inattention to infant/child needs ■ Inappropriate care taking behaviors (toilet training, sleep/rest, feeding) ■ History of child abuse or abandonment by primary caretaker ○ Lack of parental attachment behaviors:

> Inappropriate visual, tactile, auditory stimulation
> Negative identification of infant/child's characteristics
> Negative attachment of meanings to infant/child characteristics
> Noncompliance with health appointments for self and/or infant/child

○ Inappropriate or inconsistent discipline practices ○ Frequent accidents/illness ○ Growth and development lag in the child ○ Child receives care from multiple caretakers without consideration for the needs of the infant/child ○ Compulsive seeking of role approval from others ○ Abandonment; runaway

Parenting, altered, risk for*

DEFINITION: The state in which a nurturing figure(s) is at risk to experience an inability to create an environment which promotes the optimum growth and development of another human being. (It is important to state as a preface to this

---

■ = critical factors/major signs and symptoms

NOTE: Information appearing in [ ] has been added by the authors to clarify and facilitate the use of nursing diagnoses.

*[**NOTE:** A risk diagnosis is not evidenced by signs and symptoms, since the problem has not yet occurred, and nursing interventions are directed at prevention. Therefore, risk factors present are noted instead.]

diagnosis that adjustment to parenting in general is a normal maturational process that elicits nursing behaviors of prevention of potential problems and health promotion.)

RISK FACTORS:[†] ○ Lack of available role model; ineffective role model ○ Lack of support between/from significant other(s) ○ Interruption in bonding process (i.e., maternal, paternal, other) ○ Mental and/or physical illness ○ Lack of knowledge ○ Limited cognitive functioning ○ Multiple pregnancies ○ Unrealistic expectation for self, infant, partner ○ Physical and psychosocial abuse of nurturing figure ○ Unmet social/emotional maturation needs of parenting figures ○ Perceived threat to own survival, physical and emotional ○ Presence of stress (financial, legal, recent crisis, cultural move [e.g., from another country, nationality]) ○ Lack of role identity ○ Lack of appropriate response of child to relationship

Perioperative Positioning, risk for injury*

DEFINITION: A state in which the client is at risk for injury as a result of the environmental conditions found in the perioperative setting.

RISK FACTORS: ○ Disorientation ○ Immobilization, muscle weakness ○ Sensory/perceptual disturbances due to anesthesia ○ Obesity ○ Emaciation ○ Edema

Peripheral Neurovascular dysfunction, risk for*

DEFINITION: A state in which an individual is at risk of experiencing a disruption in circulation, sensation, or motion of an extremity.

RISK FACTORS: ○ Fractures ○ Mechanical compression, e.g., tourniquet, cast, brace, dressing, or restraint ○ Orthopedic surgery ○ Trauma ○ Immobilization ○ Burns ○ Vascular obstruction

Personal Identity, disturbance

DEFINITION: Inability to distinguish between self and nonself.

RELATED FACTORS: To be developed by NANDA ○ [Organic brain syndrome] ○ [Poor ego differentiation, as in schizophrenia] ○ [Panic/dissociative states] ○ [Biochemical body change]

DEFINING CHARACTERISTICS: To be developed by NANDA

  SUBJECTIVE: ○ [Confusion about sense of self, purpose or direction in life, sexual identification/preference]

■ = critical factors/major signs and symptoms

NOTE: Information appearing in [ ] has been added by the authors to clarify and facilitate the use of nursing diagnoses.

*[**NOTE:** A risk diagnosis is not evidenced by signs and symptoms, since the problem has not yet occurred, and nursing interventions are directed at prevention. Therefore, risk factors present are noted instead.]

[†] NANDA has identified these as Related Factors. However, we believe they are Risk Factors. The Risk Factors originally identified by NANDA for this diagnosis are actually the Defining Characteristics for the actual nursing diagnosis "Parenting, altered." We believe that the presence of the "Risk Factors" originally identified by NANDA indicated an actual problem.

OBJECTIVE: ○ [Difficulty in making decisions] ○ [Poorly differentiated ego boundaries] ○ [See ND Anxiety, Panic State]

Physical Mobility, impaired [specify level]

DEFINITION: A state in which the individual experiences a limitation of ability for independent physical movement.

RELATED FACTORS: ○ Intolerance to activity/decreased strength and endurance ○ Pain/discomfort ○ Neuromuscular/musculoskeletal impairment ○ Perceptual/cognitive impairment ○ Depression/severe anxiety ○ [Restrictive therapies/safety precautions, e.g., bedrest, limb immobilization] ○ [Effects of therapies, e.g., medication]

DEFINING CHARACTERISTICS:

SUBJECTIVE: ○ Reluctance to attempt movement ○ [Reports of pain/discomfort on movement]

OBJECTIVE: ○ Inability to purposefully move within the physical environment, including bed mobility, transfer, and ambulation ○ Impaired coordination ○ Limited range of motion ○ Decreased muscle strength, control, and/or mass ○ Imposed restrictions of movement, including mechanical, medical protocol

○ Suggested Functional Level Classification:

   0=Completely independent
   1=Requires use of equipment or device
   2=Requires help from another person for assistance, supervision, or teaching
   3=Requires help from another person and equipment device
   4=Dependent, does not participate in activity (Code adapted from E. Jones, et al. [November 1974]. Patient classification for long-term care: User's manual, HEW, Publication No. HRA-74-3107.)

Poisoning, risk for*

DEFINITION: Accentuated risk of accidental exposure to or ingestion of drugs or dangerous products in dosages sufficient to cause poisoning. [Adverse effects of prescribed medication/drug use.]

RISK FACTORS:

INTERNAL (INDIVIDUAL): ○ Reduced vision ○ Lack of safety or drug education ○ Lack of proper precaution ○ Insufficient finances ○ Verbalization of occupational setting without adequate safeguards ○ Cognitive or emotional difficulties ○ [Age, e.g., young child, elderly] ○ [Chronic disease state, disability] ○ [Careless behaviors, attitudes, habits, belief systems]

■ = critical factors/major signs and symptoms

NOTE: Information appearing in [ ] has been added by the authors to clarify and facilitate the use of nursing diagnoses.

*[**NOTE:** A risk diagnosis is not evidenced by signs and symptoms, since the problem has not yet occurred, and nursing interventions are directed at prevention. Therefore, risk factors present are noted instead.]

EXTERNAL (ENVIRONMENTAL): ○ Large supplies of drugs in house ○ Dangerous products placed or stored within the reach of children or confused persons ○ Flaking, peeling paint or plaster in presence of young children ○ Paint, lacquer, and so on, in poorly ventilated areas or without effective protection ○ [Unsafe stoves, heaters; lack of smoke detectors] ○ Medicines stored in unlocked cabinets accessible to children or confused persons ○ Availability of illicit drugs potentially contaminated by poisonous additives ○ Chemical contamination of food and water ○ Unprotected contact with heavy metals or chemicals ○ Presence of poisonous vegetation ○ Presence of atmospheric pollutants

Post-Trauma Response [specify stage]

DEFINITION: The state of an individual experiencing a sustained painful response to an overwhelming traumatic event.

RELATED FACTORS: ○ Disasters [e.g., floods, earthquakes, tornadoes, airplane crashes], wars, epidemics, rape, assault, torture, catastrophic illness, or accident, [being held hostage].

DEFINING CHARACTERISTICS:

SUBJECTIVE: ■ Reexperience of the traumatic event which may be identified in cognitive, affective, and/or sensory motor activities (flashbacks, intrusive thoughts, repetitive dreams or nightmares, excessive verbalization of the traumatic event, verbalization of survival guilt or guilt about behavior required for survival) ○ [Somatic reactions: chronic pains, nausea, changes in appetite, skeletal/muscle tension, exaggerated startle response, sensitivity to noise, insomnia, headaches, dizziness, unsteadiness, chronic fatigue and easy fatigability, sleep disturbance]

OBJECTIVE: ○ Psychic/emotional numbness (impaired interpretation of reality, confusion, dissociation or amnesia, vagueness about traumatic event, constricted affect) ○ Altered lifestyle (self-destructiveness such as substance abuse, suicide attempt or other acting out behavior, difficulty with interpersonal relationships; [loss of interest in usual activities, detachment, loss of feeling of intimacy/sexuality]; development of phobia regarding trauma, poor impulse control/irritability and explosiveness) ○ [Disturbance of mood (e.g., depression, anxiety, embarrassment, fear, humiliation, self-blame, low self-esteem), fear of violence toward self or others] ○ [Cognitive disruption: confusion, loss of memory/concentration, indecisiveness] ○ [Social reactions: Dependence on others, work/school failure, avoidance of close relationships, social isolation]
[Stages:

Acute subtype: Begins within 6 months and does not last longer than 6 months
Chronic subtype: Lasts more than 6 months
Delayed subtype: Period of latency of 6 months or more before onset of symptoms]

■ = critical factors/major signs and symptoms

NOTE: Information appearing in [ ] has been added by the authors to clarify and facilitate the use of nursing diagnoses.

Powerlessness [specify level]

DEFINITION: Perception that one's own action will not significantly affect an outcome; a perceived lack of control over a current situation or immediate happening.

RELATED FACTORS: ○ Healthcare environment [e.g., loss of privacy, personal possessions, control over therapies] ○ Interpersonal interaction [e.g., misuse of power, force; abusive relationships] ○ Illness-related regimen [e.g., chronic/debilitating conditions] ○ Lifestyle of helplessness [e.g., repeated failures, dependency]

DEFINING CHARACTERISTICS

SUBJECTIVE

Severe: ○ Verbal expressions of having no control or influence over situation, outcome, or self-care ○ Depression over physical deterioration which occurs despite patient compliance with regimens

Moderate: ○ Expressions of dissatisfaction and frustration over inability to perform previous tasks and/or activities ○ Expression of doubt regarding role performance ○ Reluctance to express true feelings; fearing alienation from caregivers

Low: ○ Expressions of uncertainty about fluctuating energy levels

OBJECTIVE

Severe: ○ Apathy; [withdrawn, resigned, crying] ○ [Anger]

Moderate: ○ Does not monitor progress ○ Nonparticipation in care or decision-making when opportunities are provided ○ Dependence on others that may result in irritability, resentment, anger, and guilt ○ Inability to seek information regarding care ○ Does not defend self-care practices when challenged ○ Passivity

Low: ○ Passivity

Protection, altered

DEFINITION: The state in which an individual experiences a decrease in the ability to guard the self from internal or external threats such as illness or injury.

RELATED FACTORS: ○ Extremes of age ○ Inadequate nutrition ○ Alcohol abuse ○ Abnormal blood profiles (leukopenia, thrombocytopenia, anemia, coagulation) ○ Drug therapies (antineoplastic, corticosteroid, immune, anticoagulant, thrombolytic) ○ Treatments (surgery, radiation) ○ Diseases (such as cancer and immune disorders)

DEFINING CHARACTERISTICS:

SUBJECTIVE: ○ Neurosensory alterations ○ Chilling ○ Itching ○ Insomnia; fatigue; weakness ○ Anorexia

OBJECTIVE: ■ Deficient immunity ■ Impaired healing ■ Altered clotting ■ Maladaptive stress response ○ Perspiring ○ Dyspnea; cough ○ Restlessness; immobility ○ Disorientation ○ Pressure sores

---

■ = critical factors/major signs and symptoms

NOTE: Information appearing in [ ] has been added by the authors to clarify and facilitate the use of nursing diagnoses.

[**Note:** The purpose of this diagnosis seems to be to provide for the combining of multiple diagnoses under a single heading for ease of planning care when a number of variables may be present, such as:

Extremes of age: Concern may be about Body Temperature, altered, risk for/Thermoregulation, or Thought Process, altered/Sensory-Perceptual alterations; (specify): visual, auditory, kinesthetic, gustatory, tactile, olfactory, as well as Trauma, risk for, Suffocation, risk for, or Poisoning, risk for.

Abnormal blood profile: Suggests possibility of Fluid Volume deficit, Tissue Perfusion, impaired; Gas Exchange, impaired; or Infection, risk for.

Inadequate Nutrition: Brings up issues of Nutrition, altered, less than/more than body requirements; Infection, risk for; Thought Processes, altered; or Trauma, risk for.

Alcohol Abuse: May be situational or chronic with problems ranging from Breathing Patterns, ineffective; Cardiac Output, decreased; and Fluid Volume deficit to Nutrition, less/more than body requirements; Infection, risk for; Trauma, risk for; or Thought Processes, altered.]

Rape-Trauma Syndrome [specify]

DEFINITION: Forced, violent sexual penetration against the victim's will and consent. The trauma syndrome that develops from this attack or attempted attack includes an acute phase of disorganization of the victim's lifestyle and a long-term process of reorganization of lifestyle. [This syndrome includes the following three subcomponents: Rape trauma (A); Compound reaction (B), and Silent reaction (C)]. [Note: While attacks are most often directed toward women, men also may be victims.]

RELATED FACTORS: ○ [Victim of actual/attempted forced sexual penetration]

DEFINING CHARACTERISTICS

A: RAPE TRAUMA

Acute Phase: ○ Emotional reactions (anger, embarrassment, fear of physical violence and death, humiliation, revenge, self-blame) ○ Multiple physical symptoms (gastrointestinal irritability, genitourinary discomfort, muscle tension, sleep pattern disturbance)

Long-term Phase ○ Changes in lifestyle (change in residence; dealing with repetitive nightmares and phobias; seeking family support; seeking social network support)

B: COMPOUND REACTION: ○ All defining characteristics listed under rape trauma; in addition:

Acute Phase: ○ Reactivated symptoms of such previous conditions, i.e., physical/psychiatric illness ○ Reliance on alcohol and/or drugs

C: SILENT REACTIONS: ○ Abrupt changes in relationships with men ○ Increase in nightmares ○ Increasing anxiety during interview, that is, blocking of associations, long periods of silence, minor stuttering, physical distress ○ Pro-

---

■ = critical factors/major signs and symptoms

NOTE: Information appearing in [ ] has been added by the authors to clarify and facilitate the use of nursing diagnoses.

nounced changes in sexual behavior ○ No verbalization of the occurrence of rape ○ Sudden onset of phobic reactions

Relocation Stress Syndrome

DEFINITION: Physiologic and/or psychosocial disturbances as a result of transfer from one environment to another.

RELATED FACTORS: ○ Past, concurrent, and recent losses ○ Losses involved with decision to move ○ Feeling of powerlessness ○ Lack of adequate support system ○ Little or no preparation for the move ○ Moderate to high degree of environmental change ○ History and types of previous transfers ○ Impaired psychosocial health status ○ Decreased physical health status

DEFINING CHARACTERISTICS

SUBJECTIVE: ■ Anxiety ■ Apprehension ■ Depression ■ Loneliness ○ Verbalization of unwillingness to relocate ○ Sleep disturbance ○ Change in eating habits ○ Increased verbalization of needs ○ Gastrointestinal disturbances ○ Insecurity ○ Lack of trust ○ Verbalization of being concerned/upset about transfer ○ Unfavorable comparison of post-/pretransfer staff

OBJECTIVE: ■ Change in environment/location ■ Increased confusion (elderly population [/cognitively impaired]) ○ Dependency ○ Sad affect ○ Vigilance ○ Weight change ○ Withdrawal

Role Performance, altered

DEFINITION: Disruption in the way one perceives one's role performance.

RELATED FACTORS: To be developed by NANDA ○ [Crisis:] [Situational, (e.g. male head of the household is in a passive, dependent patient role), absence of role model, transitions, conflicts] ○ [Developmental (age, values/beliefs)] ○ [Health-illness (e.g., chronic illness), perceptual problems]

DEFINING CHARACTERISTICS

SUBJECTIVE: ○ Change in self-perception of role ○ Denial of role ○ Lack of knowledge of role

OBJECTIVE: ○ Change in others' perception of role ○ Change in usual patterns or responsibility ○ Conflict in roles ○ Change in physical capacity to resume role ○ [Failure to assume role]

Self Care deficit (specify): feeding, bathing/hygiene, dressing/grooming, toileting

DEFINITION: A state in which the individual experiences an impaired ability to perform or complete feeding, bathing/hygiene, dressing/grooming, or toilet-

---

■ = critical factors/major signs and symptoms

NOTE: Information appearing in [ ] has been added by the authors to clarify and facilitate the use of nursing diagnoses.

ing activities for oneself [on a temporary, permanent, or progressing basis.] [**Note:** Self Care may also be expanded to include the practices used by the patient to promote health, the individual responsibility for self, a way of thinking. Refer to Home Maintenance Management, impaired; Health Maintenance, altered.]

RELATED FACTORS: ○ Intolerance to activity; decreased strength and endurance ○ Neuromuscular/musculoskeletal impairment ○ Depression; severe anxiety ○ Pain, discomfort ○ Perceptual or cognitive impairment ○ Impaired transfer ability ○ Impaired mobility status (toileting)

DEFINING CHARACTERISTICS

a. Self-Feeding deficit (levels 0 to 4)†
   ○ Inability to bring food from a receptacle to the mouth
b. Self-Bathing/Hygiene deficit (levels 0 to 4)†
   Inability to: ■ Wash body or body parts ○ Obtain or get to water source ○ Regulate temperature or flow
c. Self-Dressing/Grooming deficit (levels 0 to 4)†
   Impaired ability to: ■ Put on or take off necessary items of clothing ○ Obtain or replace articles of clothing ○ Fasten clothing ○ Maintain appearance at a satisfactory level
d. Self-Toileting deficit (levels 0 to 4)†
   Unable to: ■ Get to toilet or commode ■ Manipulate clothing for toileting ■ Sit on or rise from toilet or commode ■ Carry out proper toilet hygiene ○ Flush toilet or empty commode

† Refer to ND Physical Mobility, impaired, for definition of levels.

Self Esteem, chronic low

DEFINITION: Longstanding negative self-evaluation/feelings about self or self-capabilities ○ [Fixation in earlier level of development]

RELATED FACTORS: ○ [Continual negative evaluation of self/capabilities during childhood] ○ [Personal vulnerability] ○ [Life choices perpetuating failure] ○ [Feelings of abandonment by SO]

DEFINING CHARACTERISTICS

SUBJECTIVE: Longstanding or chronic: ■ Self-negating verbalization ■ Expressions of shame/guilt ■ Evaluates self as unable to deal with events ■ Rationalizes away/rejects positive feedback and exaggerates negative feedback about self

OBJECTIVE: ■ Longstanding or chronic hesitancy to try new things/situations ○ Frequent lack of success in work or other life events ○ Overly conforming, dependent on others' opinions ○ Excessively seeks reassurance ○ Lack of eye contact ○ Nonassertive/passive; indecisive

---

■ = critical factors/major signs and symptoms

NOTE: Information appearing in [ ] has been added by the authors to clarify and facilitate the use of nursing diagnoses.

Self Esteem disturbance

DEFINITION: Negative self-evaluation/feelings about self or self-capabilities which may be directly or indirectly expressed. [This is a human need for survival.]

RELATED FACTORS: ○ [Unsatisfactory parent-child relationship] ○ [Unrealistic expectations (on the part of self and others)] ○ [Unmet dependency needs] ○ Absent, erratic, or inconsistent parental discipline] ○ [Dysfunctional family system] ○ [Child/sexual abuse or neglect] ○ [Underdeveloped ego and punitive superego, retarded ego development] ○ [Negative role models] ○ [Disorganized or chaotic environments] ○ [Extreme poverty] ○ [Lack of positive feedback, repeated negative feedback resulting in diminished self-worth] ○ [Perceived/numerous failures (learned helplessness); "Failure" at life events, e.g., loss of job, divorce] ○ [Impaired cognition fostering negative view of self] ○ [Aging]

DEFINING CHARACTERISTICS

SUBJECTIVE: ○ Self-negating verbalization ○ Evaluates self as unable to deal with events ○ Expressions of shame/guilt ○ Rationalizes away/rejects positive feedback and exaggerates negative feedback about self ○ [Inability to accept positive reinforcement]

OBJECTIVE: ○ Hesitant to try new things/situations ○ Hypersensitive to slight or criticism ○ Grandiosity ○ Denial of problems obvious to others ○ Projection of blame/responsibility for problems ○ Rationalizing personal failures ○ [Not taking responsibility for self-care (self-neglect)] ○ [Lack of follow-through] ○ [Nonparticipation in therapy] ○ [Self-destructive behavior] ○ [Lack of eye contact]

Self Esteem, situational low

DEFINITION: Negative self-evaluation/feelings about self which develop in response to a loss or change in an individual who previously had a positive self-evaluation.

RELATED FACTORS: ○ ["Failure" at life events, (e.g., loss of job, relationship problems, divorce)] ○ [Feelings of abandonment by SO] ○ [Maturational transitions, adolescence, aging] ○ [Perceived loss of control in some aspect of life] ○ [Loss of independent functioning] ○ [Loss of capacity for remembering] ○ [Loss of capability for effective verbal communication]

DEFINING CHARACTERISTICS

SUBJECTIVE: ■ Episodic occurrence of negative self-appraisal in response to life events in a person with a previous positive self-evaluation ■ Verbalization of negative feelings about the self (helplessness, uselessness) ○ Self-negating verbalizations; expressions of shame/guilt ○ Evaluates self as unable to handle situations/events

OBJECTIVE: ○ Difficulty making decisions

■ = critical factors/major signs and symptoms

NOTE: Information appearing in [ ] has been added by the authors to clarify and facilitate the use of nursing diagnoses.

Self-Mutilation, risk for*

DEFINITION: A state in which an individual is at risk to perform an act upon the self to injure, not kill, which produces tissue damage and tension relief.

RISK FACTORS ○ Groups at risk: Clients with borderline personality disorder, especially females 16 to 25 years of age; clients in psychotic state—frequently males in young adulthood; emotionally disturbed and/or battered children; mentally retarded and autistic children; clients with a history of self-injury, physical, emotional or sexual abuse ○ Inability to cope with increased psychological/physiological tension in a healthy manner ○ Feelings of depression, rejection, self-hatred, separation anxiety, guilt, and depersonalization ○ Fluctuating emotions ○ Command hallucinations ○ Need for sensory stimuli ○ Parental emotional deprivation ○ Dysfunctional family

Sensory-Perceptual alterations (specify): visual, auditory, kinesthetic, gustatory, tactile, olfactory

DEFINITION: A state in which an individual experiences a change in the amount or patterning of incoming stimuli accompanied by a diminished, exaggerated, distorted, or impaired response to such stimuli.

RELATED FACTORS: ○ Altered environmental stimuli, excessive or insufficient: [Therapeutically restricted environments, e.g., isolation, intensive care, bed rest, traction, confining illnesses, incubator ○ Socially restricted environment (e.g., institutionalization, homebound, aging, chronic illness/dying, infant deprivation), stigmatized (e.g., mentally ill/retarded/handicapped), bereaved ○ Excessive noise level, e.g., work environment, patient's immediate environment (intensive care unit with support machinery, etc.)] ○ Altered sensory reception, transmission, and/or integration: [Neurologic disease, trauma, or deficit; altered status of sense organs ○ Inability to communicate, understand, speak, or respond; sleep deprivation; pain, (phantom limb)] ○ Chemical alterations: Endogenous (electrolyte), [elevated BUN, elevated ammonia, hypoxia]; exogenous (drugs [central nervous system stimulants or depressants, mind-altering drugs], etc.) ○ Psychological stress [narrowed perceptual fields caused by anxiety]

DEFINING CHARACTERISTICS

SUBJECTIVE: ○ Anxiety [panic state] ○ Indication of body image alteration ○ Reported change in sensory acuity [e.g., photosensitivity, hypo/hyperesthesias, diminished/altered sense of taste, inability to tell position of body parts (proprioception)] ○ [Pain]

OBJECTIVE: ○ Measured change in sensory acuity ○ Change in problem-solving abilities, [lack of/poor concentration] ○ Altered abstraction/conceptualiza-

---

■ = critical factors/major signs and symptoms

NOTE: Information appearing in [ ] has been added by the authors to clarify and facilitate the use of nursing diagnoses.

*[**NOTE:** A risk diagnosis is not evidenced by signs and symptoms, since the problem has not yet occurred, and nursing interventions are directed at prevention. Therefore, risk factors present are noted instead.]

tion, [disordered thought sequencing] ○ Disoriented in time, in place, or with persons ○ Altered communication patterns ○ Change in usual response to stimuli, [rapid mood swings, exaggerated emotional responses] ○ Changes in behavior pattern ○ Apathy ○ Restlessness, irritability ○ [Bizarre thinking] ○ [Motor incoordination; altered sense of balance/falls, e.g., Meniere's syndrome] Other possible defining characteristics:

SUBJECTIVE: ○ Reports of fatigue

OBJECTIVE: ○ Change in muscular tension ○ Alteration in posture ○ Inappropriate responses ○ Hallucinations

Sexual dysfunction

DEFINITION: The state in which an individual experiences a change in sexual function that is viewed as unsatisfying, unrewarding, or inadequate.

RELATED FACTORS: ○ Biopsychosocial alteration of sexuality: ○ Ineffectual or absent role models ○ Vulnerability ○ Misinformation or lack of knowledge ○ Physical abuse ○ Values conflict ○ Lack of privacy ○ Altered body structure or function (pregnancy, recent childbirth, drugs, surgery, anomalies, disease process, trauma, radiation, [loss of sexual desire, disruption of sexual response pattern such as premature ejaculation, dyspareunia]) ○ Psychosocial abuse, e.g., harmful relationships ○ Lack of significant other

DEFINING CHARACTERISTICS

SUBJECTIVE: ○ Verbalization of problem ○ Actual or perceived limitation imposed by disease and/or therapy ○ Inability to achieve desired satisfaction ○ Alterations in achieving perceived sex role ○ Conflicts involving values ○ Alterations in achieving sexual satisfaction ○ Seeking of confirmation of desirability

OBJECTIVE: ○ Alteration in relationship with significant other ○ Change of interest in self and others

Sexuality Patterns, altered

DEFINITION: The state in which an individual expresses concern regarding his/her sexuality.

RELATED FACTORS: ○ Knowledge/skill deficit about alternative responses to health-related transitions, altered body function or structure, illness or medical treatment ○ Lack of privacy ○ Lack of significant other ○ Ineffective or absent role models ○ Conflicts with sexual orientation or variant preferences ○ Fear of pregnancy or of acquiring a sexually transmitted disease ○ Impaired relationship with a significant other

---

■ = critical factors/major signs and symptoms

NOTE: Information appearing in [ ] has been added by the authors to clarify and facilitate the use of nursing diagnoses.

DEFINING CHARACTERISTICS

SUBJECTIVE: ▪ Reported difficulties, limitations, or changes in sexual behaviors or activities.

Skin Integrity, impaired

DEFINITION: A state in which the individual's skin is adversely altered. [An interruption in the integumentary system, the largest, multifunctional organ of the body.]

RELATED FACTORS

EXTERNAL (ENVIRONMENTAL): ○ Hyperthermia or hypothermia ○ Chemical substance ○ Radiation ○ Physical immobilization ○ Humidity ○ Mechanical factors (shearing forces, pressure, restraint), [trauma: injury/surgery] ○ [Excretions/secretions]

INTERNAL (SOMATIC): ○ Medication ○ Altered nutritional state (obesity, emaciation); metabolic state; circulation; sensation; pigmentation ○ Skeletal prominence ○ Developmental factors ○ Alterations in turgor (change in elasticity) ○ Immunological deficit ○ [Excretions/secretions] ○ [Psychogenic] ○ [Presence of edema]

DEFINING CHARACTERISTICS

SUBJECTIVE: ○ [Reports of itching, pain, numbness of affected/surrounding area]

OBJECTIVE: ○ Disruption of skin surface ○ Destruction of skin layers ○ Invasion of body structures

Skin Integrity, impaired, risk for*

DEFINITION: A state in which the individual's skin is at risk of being adversely altered.

RISK FACTORS

EXTERNAL (ENVIRONMENTAL): ○ Chemical substance ○ Hypothermia or hyperthermia ○ Radiation ○ Physical immobilization ○ Excretions and secretions ○ Humidity ○ Mechanical factors (shearing forces, pressure, restraint)

INTERNAL (SOMATIC): ○ Medication ○ Altered nutritional state (obesity, emaciation); metabolic state; circulation; sensation; pigmentation ○ Skeletal prominence ○ Developmental factors ○ Alterations in skin turgor (change in elasticity) ○ Psychogenic ○ Immunologic ○ [Presence of edema]

▪ = critical factors/major signs and symptoms

NOTE: Information appearing in [ ] has been added by the authors to clarify and facilitate the use of nursing diagnoses.

*[**NOTE:** A risk diagnosis is not evidenced by signs and symptoms, since the problem has not yet occurred, and nursing interventions are directed at prevention. Therefore, risk factors present are noted instead.]

Sleep Pattern disturbance

DEFINITION: Disruption of sleep time which causes patient discomfort or interferes with desired lifestyle.

RELATED FACTORS

SENSORY ALTERATIONS: ○ Internal (illness, [pain]; psychologic stress [anxiety, depression]; [inactivity]) ○ External (environment changes [including change of work shift, hospital routine]; social cues [e.g., demands of caring for others])

DEFINING CHARACTERISTICS

SUBJECTIVE: ▪ Verbal reports of: Difficulty in falling asleep ▪ Not feeling well rested ▪ Awakening earlier or later than desired ▪ Interrupted sleep ○ [Falls asleep during activities]

OBJECTIVE: ○ Changes in behavior and performance (increasing irritability, disorientation, listlessness, restlessness, lethargy) ○ Physical signs (mild, fleeting nystagmus, ptosis of eyelid, slight hand tremor, expressionless face, dark circles under eyes, changes in posture, frequent yawning) ○ Thick speech with mispronunciation and incorrect words

Social Interaction, impaired

DEFINITION: The state in which an individual participates in an insufficient or excessive quantity or ineffective quality of social exchange.

RELATED FACTORS: ○ Knowledge/skill deficit about ways to enhance mutuality ○ Communication barriers [including head injury, stroke, other neurologic conditions affecting ability to communicate] ○ Self-concept disturbance ○ Absence of available significant other(s) or peers ○ Limited physical mobility [e.g., neuromuscular disease] ○ Therapeutic isolation ○ Sociocultural dissonance ○ Environmental barriers ○ Altered thought processes

DEFINING CHARACTERISTICS

SUBJECTIVE: ▪ Verbalized discomfort in special situations ▪ Verbalized inability to receive or communicate a satisfying sense of belonging, caring, interest, or shared history ○ Family report of change of style or pattern of interaction

OBJECTIVE: ▪ Observed discomfort in social situations ▪ Observed inability to receive or communicate a satisfying sense of belonging, caring, interest, or shared history ▪ Observed use of unsuccessful social interaction behaviors ▪ Dysfunctional interaction with peers, family, and/or others

Social Isolation

DEFINITION: Aloneness experienced by the individual and perceived as imposed by others and as a negative or threatened state.

▪ = critical factors/major signs and symptoms

NOTE: Information appearing in [ ] has been added by the authors to clarify and facilitate the use of nursing diagnoses.

RISK FACTORS: Factors contributing to the absence of satisfying personal relationships, such as: ○ Delay in accomplishing developmental tasks ○ Immature interests ○ Alterations in mental status ○ Altered state of wellness ○ Alterations in physical appearance ○ Unaccepted social behavior/values ○ Inadequate personal resources ○ Inability to engage in satisfying personal relationships ○ [Traumatic incidents or events]

DEFINING CHARACTERISTICS

SUBJECTIVE: Expresses: ■ Feeling of aloneness imposed by others ■ Feelings of rejection ○ Values acceptable to subculture but unacceptable to the dominant cultural group ○ Inability to meet expectations of others ○ Experiencing feelings of difference from others ○ Inadequacy in or absence of significant purpose in life ○ Interests inappropriate to developmental age/stage ○ Insecurity in public

OBJECTIVE: ■ Absence of supportive significant other(s)—family, friends, group ○ Sad, dull affect ○ Inappropriate or immature interests/activities for developmental age/stage ○ Projects hostility in voice, behavior ○ Evidence of physical/mental handicap or altered state of wellness ○ Uncommunicative, withdrawn, no eye contact ○ Preoccupation with own thoughts, repetitive, meaningless actions ○ Seeks to be alone, or exists in subculture ○ Shows behavior unaccepted by dominant cultural group

Spiritual Distress (distress of the human spirit)

DEFINITION: Disruption in the life principle which pervades a person's entire being and which integrates and transcends one's biologic and psychosocial nature.

RELATED FACTORS: ○ Separation from religious and cultural ties ○ Challenged belief and value system, (e.g., due to moral/ethical implications of therapy, due to intense suffering)

DEFINING CHARACTERISTICS

SUBJECTIVE: ■ Expresses concern with meaning of life/death and/or belief systems ○ Verbalizes inner conflict about beliefs; concern about relationship with deity; does not experience that God is forgiving ○ Questions moral/ethical implications of therapeutic regimen ○ Description of nightmares/sleep disturbances ○ Anger toward God [as defined by the person]; displacement of anger toward religious representatives ○ Questions meaning of suffering ○ Questions meaning of own existence ○ Seeks spiritual assistance ○ Unable to choose [or chooses not to] participate in usual religious practices ○ [Regards illness as punishment] ○ [Unable to accept self; engages in self-blame] ○ [Description of somatic complaints]

OBJECTIVE: ○ Alteration in behavior or mood evidenced by anger, crying, withdrawal, preoccupation, anxiety, hostility, apathy, and so on ○ Gallows humor

---

■ = critical factors/major signs and symptoms

NOTE: Information appearing in [ ] has been added by the authors to clarify and facilitate the use of nursing diagnoses.

Spiritual Well-Being, enhanced potential for

DEFINITION: Spiritual well-being is the process of an individual's developing/unfolding of mystery through harmonious interconnectedness that springs from inner strengths.

RELATED FACTORS: [None listed]

DEFINING CHARACTERISTICS

SUBJECTIVE: ○ Inner strengths: A sense of awareness, self-consciousness, sacred source, unifying force, inner core, and transcendence ○ Unfolding mystery: one's experience about life's purpose and meaning, mystery, uncertainty, and struggles ○ Harmonious interconnectedness: relatedness, connectedness, harmony with self, others, higher power/God, and the environment

Spontaneous Ventilation, inability to sustain

DEFINITION: A state in which the response pattern of decreased energy reserves results in an individual's inability to maintain breathing adequate to support life.

RELATED FACTORS: ○ Metabolic factors ○ Respiratory muscle fatigue

DEFINING CHARACTERISTICS

SUBJECTIVE: ■ Dyspnea ○ Apprehensive

OBJECTIVE: ■ Increased metabolic rate ○ Increased restlessness ○ Increased use of accessory muscles ○ Decreased tidal volume ○ Increased heart rate ○ Decreased Po_2 ○ Decreased Pco_2 ○ Decreased cooperation ○ Decreased Sao_2

Suffocation, risk for*

DEFINITION: Accentuated risk of accidental suffocation (inadequate air available for inhalation).

RISK FACTORS

INTERNAL (INDIVIDUAL): ○ Reduced olfactory sensation ○ Reduced motor abilities ○ Lack of safety education; precautions ○ Cognitive or emotional difficulties [e.g., altered consciousness] ○ Disease or injury process

EXTERNAL (ENVIRONMENTAL): ○ Pillow/propped bottle placed in an infant's crib ○ Pacifier hung around infant's head ○ Children playing with plastic bags or inserting small objects into their mouths or noses ○ Children left unattended in bathtubs or pools ○ Discarded or unused refrigerators or freezers without removed doors ○ Vehicle warming in closed garage ○ Household gas leaks ○ Smoking in bed ○ Use of fuel-burning heaters not vented to outside ○ Low-strung clothesline ○ Eating of large mouthfuls [or pieces] of food

---

■ = critical factors/major signs and symptoms

NOTE: Information appearing in [ ] has been added by the authors to clarify and facilitate the use of nursing diagnoses.

*[**NOTE:** A risk diagnosis is not evidenced by signs and symptoms, since the problem has not yet occurred, and nursing interventions are directed at prevention. Therefore, risk factors present are noted instead.]

Swallowing, impaired

DEFINITION: The state in which an individual has decreased ability to voluntarily pass fluids and/or solids from the mouth to the stomach.

RELATED FACTORS: ○ Neuromuscular impairment (e.g., decreased or absent gag reflex, decreased strength or excursion of muscles involved in mastication [and swallowing], perceptual impairment [decreased sensation in oral cavity], facial paralysis) ○ Mechanical obstruction (e.g., edema, tracheostomy tube, tumor) ○ Fatigue ○ Limited awareness ○ Reddened, irritated oropharyngeal cavity

DEFINING CHARACTERISTICS

OBJECTIVE: ○ Observed evidence of difficulty in swallowing (e.g., stasis of food in oral cavity [pocketing/squirreling of food, food sticking], coughing/choking); [drooling, stranding phlegm, swallowing incoordination, repeated swallows, nasal regurgitation, wet/hoarse voice] ○ Evidence of aspiration, [foamy phlegm] ○ [Facial droop, difficulty chewing]

Therapeutic Regimen: Community, ineffective management

DEFINITION: A pattern of regulating and integrating into community processes programs for treatment of illness and the sequelae of illness that are unsatisfactory for meeting health-related goals.

RELATED FACTORS: [None listed]

DEFINING CHARACTERISTICS

OBJECTIVE: ○ Deficits in persons and programs to be accountable for illness care of aggregates ○ Deficits in advocates for aggregates ○ Deficits in community activities for secondary and tertiary prevention ○ Illness symptoms above the norm expected for the number and type of population ○ Number of healthcare resources are insufficient for the incidence or prevalence of illness(es) ○ Unavailable healthcare resources for illness care ○ Unexpected acceleration of illness(es)

Therapeutic Regimen: Families, ineffective management

DEFINITION: A pattern of regulating and integrating into family processes a program for treatment of illness and the sequelae of illness that is unsatisfactory for meeting specific goals.

RELATED FACTORS: ○ Complexity of healthcare system ○ Complexity of therapeutic regimen ○ Decisional conflicts ○ Economic difficulties ○ Excessive demands made on individual or family ○ Family conflicts

---

■ = critical factors/major signs and symptoms

NOTE: Information appearing in [ ] has been added by the authors to clarify and facilitate the use of nursing diagnoses.

DEFINING CHARACTERISTICS

SUBJECTIVE: ○ Verbalized desire to manage the treatment of illness and pre-vention of the sequelae ○ Verbalized difficulty with regulation/integration of one or more effects or prevention of complication ○ Verbalizes that family did not take action to reduce risk factors for progression of illness and sequelae

OBJECTIVE: ■ Inappropriate family activities for meeting the goals of a treat-ment or prevention program ○ Acceleration (expected or unexpected) of illness symptoms of a family member ○ Lack of attention to illness and its sequelae

Therapeutic Regimen: Individual, effective management

DEFINITION: A pattern of regulating and integrating into daily living a program for treatment of illness and its sequelae that is satisfactory for meeting specific health goals.

RELATED FACTORS: [None listed]

DEFINING CHARACTERISTICS

SUBJECTIVE: ○ Verbalized desire to manage the treatment of illness and pre-vention of sequelae ○ Verbalized intent to reduce risk factors for progression of illness and sequelae

OBJECTIVE: ○ Appropriate choices of daily activities for meeting the goals of a treatment or prevention program ○ Illness symptoms are within a normal range of expectation

Therapeutic Regimen: Individual, ineffective management

DEFINITION: A pattern of regulating and integrating into daily living a program for treatment of illness and the sequelae of illness that is unsatisfactory for meet-ing specific health goals.

RELATED FACTORS: ○ Complexity of healthcare system; therapeutic regimen ○ Decisional conflicts ○ Economic difficulties ○ Excessive demands made on in-dividual or family ○ Family conflict ○ Family patterns of health care ○ Inade-quate number and types of cues to action ○ Knowledge deficits ○ Mistrust of regimen and/or healthcare personnel ○ Perceived seriousness; susceptibility; barriers; benefits ○ Powerlessness ○ Social support deficits

DEFINING CHARACTERISTICS

SUBJECTIVE: Verbalized: ○ Desire to manage the treatment of illness and pre-vention of sequelae ○ Difficulty with regulation/integration of one or more pre-scribed regimens for treatment of illness and its effects on prevention of com-

---

■ = critical factors/major signs and symptoms

NOTE: Information appearing in [ ] has been added by the authors to clarify and facilitate the use of nursing diagnoses.

plications ○ Did not take action to include treatment regimens in daily routines/reduce risk factors for progression of illness and sequelae

OBJECTIVE: ■ Choice of daily living ineffective for meeting the goals of a treatment or prevention program ○ Acceleration (expected or unexpected) of illness symptoms

Thermoregulation, ineffective

DEFINITION: The state in which the individual's temperature fluctuates between hypothermia and hyperthermia.

RELATED FACTORS: ○ Trauma or illness [e.g., cerebral edema, cerebral vascular accident, intracranial surgery, or head injury] ○ Immaturity, aging [e.g., loss/absence of brown adipose tissue] ○ Fluctuating environmental temperature ○ [Changes in hypothalamic tissue causing alterations in emission of thermosensitive cells and regulation of heat loss/production] ○ [Changes in level/action of thyroxone, and catecholamines] ○ [Changes in metabolic rate/activity] ○ [Chemical reactions in contracting muscles]

DEFINING CHARACTERISTICS

OBJECTIVE: ■ Fluctuations in body temperature above or below the normal range (see also major and minor characteristics present in hypothermia and hyperthermia)

Thought Processes, altered

DEFINITION: A state in which an individual experiences a disruption in cognitive operations and activities.

RELATED FACTORS: To be developed by NANDA ○ [Physiological changes, aging, hypoxia, head injury, malnutrition, infections] ○ [Sleep deprivation] ○ [Psychological conflicts, emotional changes, mental disorders] ○ [Biochemical changes, medications, substance abuse]

DEFINING CHARACTERISTICS

SUBJECTIVE: ○ [Ideas of reference, hallucinations, delusions]

OBJECTIVE: ○ Inaccurate interpretation of environment ○ Memory deficit/problems, [disorientation to time, place, person, circumstances and events, loss of short-term/remote memory] ○ Hyper/hypovigilance ○ Cognitive dissonance, [decreased ability to grasp ideas, make decisions, problem-solve, reason, abstract or conceptualize, calculate] ○ Distractibility, [altered attention span] ○ Egocentricity ○ [Confabulation] ○ [Inappropriate social behavior]

OTHER POSSIBLE CHARACTERISTICS

OBJECTIVE: ○ Inappropriate/nonreality-based thinking

■ = critical factors/major signs and symptoms

NOTE: Information appearing in [ ] has been added by the authors to clarify and facilitate the use of nursing diagnoses.

Tissue Integrity, impaired

DEFINITION: A state in which an individual experiences damage to mucous membrane, or corneal, integumentary, or subcutaneous tissue.

RELATED FACTORS: ○ Altered circulation ○ Nutritional deficit/excess [metabolic, endocrine dysfunction] ○ Fluid deficit/excess ○ Knowledge deficit ○ Impaired physical mobility ○ Irritants, chemical (including body excretions; secretions, medications), [infections] ○ Thermal (temperature extremes) ○ Mechanical (pressure, shear, friction), radiation (including therapeutic radiation), [surgery]

DEFINING CHARACTERISTICS

OBJECTIVE: ■ Damaged or destroyed tissue (cornea, mucous membrane, integumentary, or subcutaneous)

Tissue Perfusion, altered, (specify): cerebral, cardiopulmonary, renal, gastrointestinal, peripheral

DEFINITION: The state in which an individual experiences a decrease in nutrition and oxygenation at the cellular level due to a deficit in capillary blood supply. [Tissue perfusion problems can exist without decreased cardiac output; however, there may be a relationship between cardiac output and tissue perfusion.]

RELATED FACTORS: ○ Interruption of flow—arterial, venous ○ Exchange problems ○ Hypervolemia; hypovolemia

DEFINING CHARACTERISTICS

[Cardiopulmonary and Peripheral]

SUBJECTIVE: ○ Claudication ○ [Angina, chest pain] ○ [Palpitations] ○ [Dyspnea] ○ [Feelings of impending doom]

OBJECTIVE: ■ Diminished/[absent] arterial pulsations ○ Skin color: ■ Pale on elevation, color does not return on lowering leg ○ Dependent, blue or purple, [or mottled] ○ Skin temperature: cold extremities ○ Skin quality: shining, lack of lanugo ○ Blood pressure changes in extremities ○ Bruits ○ Slow-growing, dry, thick brittle nails ○ Slow healing of lesions ○ Round scars covered with atrophied skin ○ Gangrene ○ [Delayed capillary refill] ○ [Changes in heart rate/rhythm] ○ [Central cyanosis, changes in arterial blood gases (ABGs)] ○ [Hemoptysis]
(Further work and development are required for the subcomponents, specifically cerebral, renal, and gastrointestinal.)

[Cerebral]

OBJECTIVE: ○ [Restlessness] ○ [Altered consciousness] ○ [Memory loss] ○ [Behavioral changes]

■ = critical factors/major signs and symptoms

NOTE: Information appearing in [ ] has been added by the authors to clarify and facilitate the use of nursing diagnoses.

[Renal]

OBJECTIVE: ○ [Decreased urinary output] ○ [Edema formation] ○ [Hypertension] ○ [Changes in laboratory values]

[Gastrointestinal]

OBJECTIVE: ○ [Pain] ○ [Nausea/vomiting] ○ [Abdominal distention] ○ [Melena]

Trauma, risk for*

DEFINITION: Accentuated risk of accidental tissue injury (e.g., wound, burn, fracture)

RISK FACTORS [INCLUDES BUT IS NOT LIMITED TO]

INTERNAL (INDIVIDUAL): ○ Weakness ○ Poor vision ○ Balancing difficulties ○ Reduced temperature and/or tactile sensation ○ Reduced large, or small, muscle coordination/hand/eye coordination ○ Lack of safety education/precautions ○ Insufficient finances to purchase safety equipment or effect repairs ○ Cognitive or emotional difficulties ○ History of previous trauma

EXTERNAL (ENVIRONMENTAL): ○ Slippery floors (e.g., wet or highly waxed) ○ Snow or ice collected on stairs, walkways ○ Unanchored rugs ○ Bathtub without hand grip or antislip equipment ○ Use of unsteady ladder or chairs ○ Entering unlighted rooms ○ Unsturdy or absent stair rails ○ Unanchored electric wires ○ Litter or liquid spills on floors or stairways ○ High beds ○ Children playing without gates at top of stairs ○ Obstructed passageways ○ Unsafe window protection in homes with young children ○ Inappropriate call-for-aid mechanisms for bed-resting client ○ Pot handles facing toward front of stove ○ Bathing in very hot water (unsupervised bathing of young children) ○ Potential igniting gas leaks ○ Delayed lighting of gas burner or oven ○ Experimenting with chemical or gasoline ○ Unscreened fires or heaters ○ Wearing plastic apron or flowing clothing around open flame ○ Children playing with matches, candles, cigarettes ○ Inadequately stored combustibles or corrosives (e.g., matches, oily rags, lye) ○ Highly flammable children's toys or clothing ○ Overloaded fuse boxes ○ Contact with rapidly moving machinery, industrial belts, or pulleys ○ Sliding on coarse bed linen or struggling within bed restraints ○ Faulty electric plugs, frayed wires, or defective appliances ○ Contact with acids or alkalis ○ Playing with fireworks or gunpowder ○ Contact with intense cold ○ Overexposure to sun, sun lamps, radiotherapy ○ Use of cracked dishware or glasses ○ Knives stored uncovered ○ Guns or ammunition stored unlocked ○ Large icicles hanging from roof ○ Exposure to dangerous machinery ○ Children playing with sharp-edged toys ○ High-crime neighborhood and vulnerable clients ○ Driving a mechanically unsafe vehicle ○ Driving after partaking of alcoholic beverages or drugs ○ Driving at excessive speeds ○ Driving without necessary visual aids ○ Children riding in the front seat of car ○ Smok-

---

■ = critical factors/major signs and symptoms

NOTE: Information appearing in [ ] has been added by the authors to clarify and facilitate the use of nursing diagnoses.

*[**NOTE:** A risk diagnosis is not evidenced by signs and symptoms, since the problem has not yet occurred, and nursing interventions are directed at prevention. Therefore, risk factors present are noted instead.]

ing in bed or near oxygen ○ Overloaded electric outlets ○ Grease waste collected on stoves ○ Use of thin or worn pot holders [or mitts] ○ Nonuse or misuse of necessary headgear for motorized cyclists [bicyclists/rollerbladers]/or young children carried on adult bicycles ○ Unsafe road or road-crossing conditions ○ Play or work near vehicle pathways (e.g., driveways, lanes, railroad tracks) ○ Nonuse or misuse of seat restraints/[unrestrained or improperly restrained children riding in car]

Unilateral Neglect

DEFINITION: A state in which an individual is perceptually unaware of and inattentive to one side of the body [and the immediate unilateral territory/space].

RELATED FACTORS: ○ Effects of disturbed perceptual abilities (e.g., [Homonymous] hemianopsia, [or visual inattention]) ○ One-sided blindness; neurologic illness or trauma ○ [Impaired cerebral blood flow]

DEFINING CHARACTERISTICS

SUBJECTIVE: ○ [Reports of feeling that part does not belong to own self]

OBJECTIVE: ■ Consistent inattention to stimuli on an affected side ○ Inadequate self-care [inability to satisfactorily perform activities of daily living] ○ [Lack of] Positioning and/or safety precautions in regard to the affected side ○ Does not look toward affected side ○ Leaves food on plate on the affected side ○ [Does not touch affected side] ○ [Failure to use the affected side of the body without being reminded to do so]

Urinary Elimination, altered

DEFINITION: The state in which an individual experiences a disturbance in urine elimination.

RELATED FACTORS: Multiple causality, including: ○ Sensory motor impairment ○ Anatomical obstruction ○ Urinary tract infection ○ Mechanical trauma ○ [Fluid/volume states] ○ [Psychogenic factors] ○ [Surgical diversion]

DEFINING CHARACTERISTICS

SUBJECTIVE: ○ Frequency ○ Hesitancy ○ Dysuria

OBJECTIVE: ○ Nocturia, [Enuresis] ○ Urgency ○ Incontinence ○ Retention

Urinary Retention [acute/chronic]

DEFINITION: The state in which the individual experiences incomplete emptying of the bladder. [High urethral pressure inhibits voiding until increased abdominal pressure causes urine to be involuntarily lost, or high urethral pressure inhibits timely/complete emptying of bladder.]

RELATED FACTORS: ○ High urethral pressure caused by weak detrusor [absent detrusor] ○ Inhibition of reflex arc ○ Strong sphincter; blockage [e.g., benign pro-

---

■ = critical factors/major signs and symptoms

NOTE: Information appearing in [ ] has been added by the authors to clarify and facilitate the use of nursing diagnoses.

static hypertrophy, perineal swelling] ∘ [Habituation of reflex arc] ∘ [Infections] ∘ [Neurologic diseases/trauma] ∘ [Use of medications with side effect of retention, e.g., atropine, belladonna, psychotropics, antihistamines, opiates]

DEFINING CHARACTERISTICS

SUBJECTIVE: ∘ Sensation of bladder fullness ∘ Dribbling ∘ Dysuria

OBJECTIVE: ▪ Bladder distention ▪ Small, frequent voiding or absence of urine output ∘ Residual urine [150 mL or more] ∘ Overflow incontinence ∘ [Reduced stream]

Ventilatory Weaning Response, dysfunctional (DVWR)

DEFINITION: A state in which a patient cannot adjust to lowered levels of mechanical ventilator support, which interrupts and prolongs the weaning process.

RELATED FACTORS

PHYSICAL: ∘ Ineffective airway clearance ∘ Sleep pattern disturbance ∘ Inadequate nutrition ∘ Uncontrolled pain or discomfort ∘ [Immobility] ∘ [Muscle weakness/fatigue, inability to control respiratory muscles]

PSYCHOLOGICAL: ∘ Knowledge deficit of the weaning process, patient role ∘ Patient perceived inefficacy about the ability to wean ∘ Decreased motivation ∘ Decreased self-esteem ∘ Anxiety: moderate, severe ∘ Fear ∘ Hopelessness ∘ Powerlessness ∘ Insufficient trust in the nurse ∘ [Unprepared for weaning attempt]

SITUATIONAL: ∘ Uncontrolled episodic energy demands or problems ∘ Inappropriate pacing of diminished ventilator support ∘ Inadequate social support ∘ Adverse environment (noisy, active environment, negative events in the room, low nurse-patient ratio, extended nurse absence from bedside, unfamiliar nursing staff) ∘ History of ventilator dependence for more than 1 week ∘ History of multiple unsuccessful weaning attempts

DEFINING CHARACTERISTICS: Responds to lowered levels of mechanical ventilator support with:

Mild DVWR

SUBJECTIVE: ∘ Expressed feelings of increased need for oxygen/breathing ∘ Queries about possible machine malfunction

OBJECTIVE: ▪ Restlessness ▪ Slight increased respiratory rate from baseline ∘ Increased concentration on breathing

Moderate DVWR

SUBJECTIVE: ∘ Apprehension

OBJECTIVE: ▪ Slight increase from baseline BP (less than 20 mm Hg) ▪ Slight increase from baseline heart rate (less than 20 bpm) ▪ Baseline increase in respiratory rate (less than 5 breaths/min) ∘ Hypervigilance to activities ∘ Inability to

---

▪ = critical factors/major signs and symptoms

NOTE: Information appearing in [ ] has been added by the authors to clarify and facilitate the use of nursing diagnoses.

respond to coaching ○ Inability to cooperate ○ Diaphoresis ○ Eye widening "wide-eyed look" ○ Decreased air entry on auscultation ○ Color changes; pale, slight cyanosis ○ Slight respiratory accessory muscle use

Severe DVWR

OBJECTIVE: ■ Agitation ■ Deterioration in ABG from current baseline ■ Increase from baseline BP (greater than 20 mm Hg) ■ Increase from baseline heart rate (greater than 20 bpm) ■ Respiratory rate increase significantly from baseline ○ Profuse diaphoresis ○ Full respiratory accessory muscle use ○ Shallow, gasping breaths ○ Paradoxical abdominal breathing ○ Discoordinated breathing with the ventilator ○ Decreased level of consciousness ○ Adventitious breath sounds, audible airway secretions ○ Cyanosis

Violence [actual]/risk for; directed at self/others*

DEFINITION: A state in which an individual experiences behaviors that can be physically harmful either to the self or others. [The "harm" can range from neglect to abuse or even death and may be psychological and/or physical.]

RELATED [/RISK] FACTORS: ○ Antisocial character ○ Catatonic/manic excitement ○ Panic states, rage reactions ○ Suicidal behavior ○ Toxic reactions to medication [including illicit drugs/alcohol] ○ Battered women [spouse abuse], child abuse ○ Organic brain syndrome; temporal lobe epilepsy ○ [Negative role modeling] ○ [Development crisis] ○ [Hormonal imbalance, e.g., PMS, postpartal depression/psychosis]

DEFINING CHARACTERISTICS [OR INDICATORS]

SUBJECTIVE: ○ **Hostile threatening verbalizations:** (boasting to or prior abuse of others) ○ [Expresses intent/desire to harm self or others, directly or indirectly]

OBJECTIVE: ○ **Body language:** (clenched fists, tense facial expressions, rigid posture, tautness indicating effort to control) ○ Increased motor activity (pacing, excitement, irritability, agitation) ○ **Overt and aggressive acts:** (goal-directed destruction of objects in environment) ○ Possession of destructive means (gun, knife, weapon) ○ Rage ○ Self-destructive behavior, active aggressive suicidal acts ○ [Acting on/] Suspicion of others, paranoid ideation, delusions, hallucinations ○ Substance abuse/withdrawal

OTHER POSSIBLE CHARACTERISTICS

SUBJECTIVE: ○ Inability to verbalize feelings ○ Fear of self or others

OBJECTIVE: ○ Provocative behavior: (argumentative, dissatisfied, overreactive, hypersensitive) ○ Vulnerable self-esteem ○ Anger ○ Repetition of verbalizations (continued complaints, requests, and demands) ○ Increasing anxiety level ○ Depression (specifically active, aggressive, suicidal acts)

■ = critical factors/major signs and symptoms

NOTE: Information appearing in [ ] has been added by the authors to clarify and facilitate the use of nursing diagnoses.

*Although a risk diagnosis does not have defining characteristics (signs and symptoms), the ones identified here can be used to denote an actual diagnosis or as indicators for risk for escalation of violence.

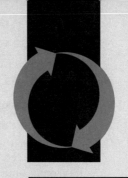

Assessment Tools

The following are suggested guides/tools for development by an individual/ institution to create data bases reflecting Diagnostic Divisions of Nursing Diagnoses in any care setting. Although the divisions are alphabetized for ease of presentation, they can be prioritized or rearranged to meet individual needs.

ADULT MEDICAL/SURGICAL ASSESSMENT TOOL

General Information

Name: _____ Age: _____ DOB: _____ Sex: _____ Race: _____
Admission Date: _____ Time: _____ From: _____
Source of Information: _____ Reliability (1–4 with 4 = very reliable): _____

ACTIVITY/REST

Subjective (Reports)

Occupation: _____ Usual
  activities/hobbies: _____
  Leisure time activities:

  _____

Feelings of boredom/
  dissatisfaction: _____
Limitations imposed by
  condition: _____
Sleep: Hours: _____ Naps: _____
  Aids: _____ Insomnia: _____
  Related to: _____
  Rested on awakening: _____
  Excessive grogginess: _____

Objective (Exhibits)

Observed response to activity:
  Cardiovascular: _____
  Respiratory: _____
Mental status (i.e., withdrawn/
  lethargic): _____
Neuro/muscular assessment:
  Muscle mass/tone: _____ Posture:
  _____ Tremors: _____ ROM: _____
  Strength: _____ Deformity: _____

CIRCULATION

Subjective (Reports)

History of: Hypertension: _____
  Heart trouble: _____
  Rheumatic fever: _____
  Ankle/leg edema: _____
  Phlebitis: _____ Slow healing: _____
  Claudication: _____ Dysreflexia:
  _____ Bleeding tendencies/
  episodes: _____ Palpitations: _____
  Syncope: _____
Extremities: Numbness: _____
  Tingling: _____
Cough/hemoptysis: _____
Change in frequency/amount of
  urine: _____
Other: _____

Objective (Exhibits)

BP: R and L:
  Lying/sit/stand: _____
  Pulse pressure: _____
  Auscultatory gap: _____
Pulse (palpation): Carotid: _____
  Temporal: _____ Jugular: _____
  Radial: _____ Femoral: _____
  Popliteal: _____ Post-tibial: _____
  Dorsalis pedis: _____
Cardiac (palpation): Thrill: _____
  Heaves: _____
Heart sounds: Rate: _____ Rhythm:
  _____ Quality: _____ Friction rub:
  _____ Murmur: _____
Breath sounds: _____
Vascular bruit: _____ Jugular vein
  distention: _____
Extremities: Temperature: _____
  Color: _____ Capillary refill: _____
  Homan's sign: _____ Varicosities:
  _____ Nail abnormalities: _____
  Edema: _____ Distribution/quality
  of hair: _____ Trophic skin
  changes: _____
Color: General: _____
  Mucous membranes: _____
  Lips: _____ Nail beds: _____
  Conjunctiva: _____ Sclera: _____
Diaphoresis: _____

EGO INTEGRITY

Subjective (Reports)

Stress factors: _____
Ways of handling stress: _____
Financial concerns: _____
Relationship status: _____
Cultural factors: _____
Religion: _____
  Practicing: _____
Lifestyle: _____ Recent
  changes: _____
Sense of connectedness/harmony
  with self: _____
Feelings of: Helplessness:
  _____ Hopelessness: _____
  Powerlessness: _____

Objective (Exhibits)

Emotional status (check those that
  apply): Calm: _____ Anxious: _____
  Angry: _____ Withdrawn: _____
  Fearful: _____ Irritable: _____
  Restive: _____ Euphoric: _____
Observed physiologic responses(s):
  _____

Changes in energy field:
  Temperature: _____ Color: _____
  Distribution: _____
  Movement: _____
  Sounds: _____

ELIMINATION

Subjective (Reports)

Usual bowel pattern: _____
Laxative use: _____
Character of stool:
_____ Last BM: _____
History of bleeding: _____
Hemorrhoids: _____
Constipation: _____ Diarrhea: _____
Usual voiding pattern: _____
Incontinence/when: _____
Urgency: _____ Frequency: _____
Retention: _____
Character of urine: _____
Pain/burning/difficulty voiding:
_____ History of kidney/bladder
disease: _____ Diuretic use: _____

Objective (Exhibits)

Abdomen: Tender: _____ Soft/firm:
_____ Palpable mass: _____ Size/
girth: _____ Bowel sounds: _____
Hemorrhoids: _____
Bladder palpable: _____ Overflow
voiding: _____
CVA tenderness: _____
Stool guaiac: _____

FOOD/FLUID

Subjective (Reports)

Usual diet (type): _____
Fat intake: _____
No. of meals daily: _____
Vitamin/food supplement use:

_____
Last meal/intake: _____
Dietary pattern/content: B: _____
L: _____ D: _____
Loss of appetite: _____
Nausea/vomiting: _____
Heartburn/indigestion: _____
Related to: _____
Relieved by: _____
Allergy/food intolerance:

_____
Mastication/swallowing problems:
_____ Dentures: _____
Usual weight: _____ Changes in
weight: _____
Diuretic use: _____

Objective (Exhibits)

Current weight: _____ Height: _____
Body build: _____
Skin turgor: _____ Mucous
membranes moist/dry: _____
Edema: General: _____ Dependent:
_____ Periorbital: _____
Ascites: _____
Jugular vein distention: _____
Thyroid enlarged: _____
Halitosis: _____ Condition of teeth/
gums: _____ Appearance of tongue:
_____ Mucous membranes: _____
Bowel sounds: _____ Breath sounds:
_____ Hernia/masses: _____
Urine S/A or Chemstix: _____
Serum glucose (Glucometer): _____

HYGIENE

Subjective (Reports)

Activities of daily living:
Independent/dependent (level):
Mobility: _____ Feeding: _____
Hygiene: _____ Dressing: _____
Toileting: _____

Objective (Exhibits)

General appearance: _____
Manner of dress: _____ Personal
habits: _____ Body odor: _____
Condition of scalp: _____
Presence of vermin: _____

Preferred time of bath: _____
Equipment/prosthetic devices
  required: _____
Assistance provided by:
  _____

NEUROSENSORY

Subjective (Reports)

Fainting spells/dizziness: _____
Headaches: Location: _____
  Frequency: _____
Tingling/numbness/weakness
  (location): _____
Stroke/brain injury (residual effects):
Seizures: _____ Type: _____
  Aura: _____ Frequency: _____
  Postictal state: _____ How
  controlled: _____
Eyes: Vision loss: _____
  Last exam: _____ Glaucoma: _____
  Cataract: _____
Ears: Hearing loss: _____
  Last exam: _____
Epistaxis: _____ Sense of smell: _____
Other: _____

Objective (Exhibits)

Mental status: _____
(note duration of change)
  Oriented/disoriented: Time: _____
  Place: _____ Person: _____
  Alert: _____ Drowsy: _____
  Lethargic: _____ Stuporous: _____
  Comatose: _____ Cooperative: _____
  Combative: _____ Delusions: _____
  Hallucinations: _____ Affect
  (describe): _____
Memory: Recent: _____ Remote: _____
Glasses: _____ Contacts: _____ Hearing
  aids: _____
Pupil shape: _____ Size/reaction: _____
  R/L: _____
Facial droop: _____ Swallowing: _____
Handgrasp/release, R/L: _____

PAIN/DISCOMFORT

Subjective (Reports)

Location, intensity (0–10 with 10
  most severe): _____
  Frequency: _____ Quality: _____
  Duration: _____ Radiation: _____
  Precipitating factors: _____
  How relieved: Associated
  symptoms: _____

Objective (Exhibits)

Facial grimacing: _____ Guarding
  affected area: _____ Emotional
  response: _____ Narrowed focus:
  _____

RESPIRATION

Subjective (Reports)

Dyspnea, related to: _____
Cough/sputum: _____
History of bronchitis: _____
  Asthma: _____ Tuberculosis: _____
  Emphysema: _____ Recurrent
  pneumonia: _____ Exposure to
  noxious fumes: _____
Smoker, packs/day: _____ No. of pack
  years: _____
Use of respiratory aids: _____
  Oxygen: _____

Objective (Exhibits)

Respiratory: Rate: _____ Depth: _____
  Symmetry: _____
Use of accessory muscles: _____
  Nasal flaring: _____
Fremitus: _____
Breath sounds: _____ Egophony: _____
Cyanosis: _____ Clubbing of
  fingers: _____
Sputum characteristics: _____
Mentation/restlessness: _____

SAFETY

Subjective (Reports)

Allergies/sensitivity: _____
    Reaction: _____
Exposure to infectious diseases:

_____

Previous alteration of immune
    system: _____ Cause: _____
History of sexually transmitted
    disease (date/type): _____
    High risk behaviors: _____
    Testing: _____
Blood transfusion/number: _____
    When: _____ Reaction: _____
    Describe: _____
Geographic areas lived in/visited:

_____

Seat belt/helmet use: _____
History of accidental injuries: _____
    Fractures/dislocations: _____
Arthritis/unstable joints: _____
    Back problems: _____
Changes in moles: _____
    Enlarged nodes: _____
Delayed healing: _____
Cognitive limitations:
    Impaired vision, hearing: _____
    Prosthesis: _____ Ambulatory
    devices _____

Objective (Exhibits)

Temperature: _____ Diaphoresis: _____
Skin integrity: _____ Scars: _____
    Rashes: _____ Lacerations: _____
    Ulcerations: _____ Ecchymosis:
    Blisters: _____ Burns: (degree/
    percent): _____ Drainage: _____
Mark location of above on diagram:

General strength: _____ Muscle tone:
    _____ Gait: _____ ROM: _____
    Paresthesia/paralysis: _____
Results of cultures: _____ Immune
    system testing: _____
Tuberculosis testing: _____

SEXUALITY [COMPONENT OF SOCIAL INTERACTION]

Subjective (Reports)

Sexually active: _____
Use of condoms: _____
Birth control method: _____
Sexual concerns/difficulties:

_____

Recent change in frequency/
    interest: _____

Female

Age at menarche: _____ Length of
    cycle: _____ Duration: _____
    Number of pads used/day: _____
    Last menstrual period: _____
Bleeding between periods: _____
Menopause: _____ Vaginal
    lubrication: _____

Objective (Exhibits)

Comfort level with subject matter:

_____

Breast exam: _____
Genital warts/lesions: _____
Discharge: _____

Vaginal discharge: _____
Surgeries: _____
Hormonal therapy/calcium use: _____
Method of birth control: _____
Practices breast self-exam: _____
Mammogram: _____ Last PAP smear:
_____

Male
Penile discharge: _____
Prostate disorder: _____
Circumcised: _____ Vasectomy: _____
Practice self-exam; Breast: _____
    Testicles: _____ Last proctoscopic/
    prostate exam: _____

Breast: _____ Penis: _____
Testicles: _____
Genital warts/lesions: _____
Discharge: _____

SOCIAL INTERACTIONS

Subjective (Reports)

Marital status: _____ Years in
    relationship: _____
    Perception of relationship: _____
    Living with: _____
    Concerns/stresses: _____
Extended family: _____ Other support
    person(s): _____
Role within family structure:

    _____

Relationship with family
    members: _____
Feelings of: Mistrust: _____
    Rejection: _____
    Unhappiness: _____
    Isolation: _____
Problems related to illness/condition:

    _____

Problems with communication: _____
    Use of communication aids: _____
Genogram: _____

Objective (Exhibits)

Speech: Clear: _____ Slurred: _____
    Unintelligible: _____ Aphasic: _____
    Unusual speech pattern/
    impairment: _____ Use of speech
    aids: _____ Laryngectomy
    present: _____
Verbal/nonverbal communication
    with family/SO(s): _____

Family interaction (behavioral)
    pattern: _____

TEACHING/LEARNING

Subjective (Reports)

Dominant language (specify):
    _____ Literate: _____
    Education level: _____ Learning
    disabilities (specify): _____
    Cognitive limitations: _____
Health beliefs/practices: _____
Special healthcare concerns (e.g.,
    impact of religious/cultural
    practices): _____

DISCHARGE PLAN CONSIDERATIONS
DRG projected mean length of
    stay: _____
Date information obtained: _____
Anticipated date of discharge: _____
Resources available: Persons:
    _____ Financial:

    _____
Community supports: _____

Health Goals: _____

Familial risk factors (indicate relationship): Diabetes: _____ Thyroid (specify): _____ Tuberculosis: _____ Heart disease: _____ Strokes: _____ High BP: _____ Epilepsy: _____ Kidney disease: _____ Cancer: _____ Mental illness: _____ Other: _____

Prescribed medications: Drug: _____ Dose: _____ Times (*circle* last dose): _____ Take regularly: _____ Purpose: _____ Side effects/problems: _____

Nonprescription drugs: OTC drugs: _____ Street drugs: _____ Tobacco: _____ Smokeless tobacco: _____

Alcohol (amount/frequency): _____

Admitting diagnosis per provider: _____

Reason for hospitalization per patient: _____

History of current complaint: _____

Patient expectations of this hospitalization: _____

Previous illnesses and/or hospitalizations/surgeries: _____

Evidence of failure to improve: _____

Last complete physical exam: _____

Groups: _____
Socialization: _____

Areas that may require alteration/assistance: Food preparation: _____ Shopping: _____ Transportation: _____ Ambulation: _____ Medication/IV therapy: _____ Treatments: _____ Wound care: _____ Supplies: _____ Self-care (specify): _____ Homemaker/maintenance (specify): _____

Physical layout of home (specify): _____

Anticipated changes in living situation after discharge: _____

Living facility other than home (specify): _____

Referrals (date, source, services): Social services: _____ Rehab services: _____ Dietary: _____ Home care: _____ Resp/O_2: _____ Equipment: _____ Supplies: _____ Other: _____

History of current complaint: _____

Patient expectations of this hospitalization: _____

Previous illness and/or hospitalizations/surgeries: _____

Evidence of failure to improve: _____

Last complete physical exam: _____

EXCERPT FROM PSYCHIATRIC NURSING ASSESSMENT TOOL

EGO INTEGRITY

Subjective (Reports)

What kind of person are you (positive/negative, etc.)? _____

What do you think of your body? _____

Objective (Exhibits)

Emotional status (check those that apply): Calm: _____ Friendly: _____ Cooperative: _____ Evasive: _____ Fearful: _____ Anxious: _____ Irritable: _____ Withdrawn: _____

How would you rate your self-esteem
(1–10; with 10 the highest)? _____
What are your moods?:
  Depressed: _____ Guilty: _____
  Unreal: _____ Ups/downs: _____
  Apathetic: _____ Separated from
  the world: _____ Detached: _____
Are you a nervous person? _____
Are your feelings easily hurt? _____
Report of stress factors: _____
Previous patterns of handling stress:

  _____
Financial concerns: _____
Relationship status: _____
Work history/Military service:

  _____
Cultural factors: _____
Religion: _____ Practicing: _____
Lifestyle: _____ Recent changes: _____
  Significant losses/changes
  (date): _____
Stages of grief/manifestations of loss:

  _____
Feelings of: Helplessness: _____
  Hopelessness: _____
  Powerlessness: _____

Restive: _____ Passive: _____
Dependent: _____ Euphoric: _____
Angry/hostile: _____ Other
  (specify): _____
Defense mechanisms: Projection: _____
  Denial: _____ Undoing: _____
  Rationalization: _____ Passive-
  aggressive: _____ Repression: _____
  Intellectualization: _____
  Somatization: _____
  Regression: _____
  Identification: _____ Introjection:
  _____ Reaction formation: _____
  Isolation: _____ Displacement: _____
  Substitution: _____
  Sublimation: _____
Consistency of behavior:

  _____
Verbal: _____ Nonverbal: _____
Characteristics of speech:

  _____
Motor behaviors: _____
Posturing: _____
Under/overactive: _____
Stereotypic: _____
Observed physiologic response(s):

  _____

NEUROSENSORY

Subjective (Reports)

Dreamlike states: _____ Walking in
  sleep: _____ Automatic writing: _____
Believe/feel you are another
  person: _____
Reports perception different than
  others: _____
Ability to follow directions: _____
Perform calculations: _____
Accomplish ADL: _____

Objective (Exhibits)

Mental Status: _____
(note duration of change)
  Oriented/disoriented: Time: _____
  Place: _____ Person: _____
Check all that apply:
  Alert: _____ Drowsy: _____
  Lethargic: _____ Stuporous: _____
  Comatose: _____ Cooperative: _____
  Combative: _____ Delusions: _____
  Hallucinations: _____ Affect
  (describe): _____
Memory: Immediate: _____ Recent:
  _____ Remote: _____
Comprehension: _____
Thought processes (assessed through
  speech): Patterns of speech
  (spontaneous/sudden silences):
  _____ Content: _____
Change in topic: _____
Delusions: _____

Hallucinations: _____ Illusions:
_____ Rate or flow: _____ Clear,
logical progression: _____
Expression: _____
Mood: _____
Affect: _____
Appropriateness: _____
Intensity: _____
Range: _____
Insight: _____
Misperceptions: _____
Attention/calculation skills:
_____ Judgment:
_____ Ability to follow
directions: _____
Problem solving: _____

EXCERPT FROM PRENATAL ASSESSMENT TOOL

SAFETY

Subjective

Allergies/Sensitivity: _____
Reaction: _____
Previous alteration of immune
system: _____ Cause _____
History of sexually transmitted
diseases/gynecologic infections
(date/type): _____ High-
risk behaviors: _____
Testing: _____
Blood transfusion/number: _____
When: _____ Reaction: _____
Describe: _____
Childhood diseases: _____
Immunization history:_____
Recent exposure to german measles:
_____ Other viral infections: _____
X-ray/radiation: _____ House
pets: _____
Previous obstetric problems:
PIH: _____ Kidney: _____
Hemorrhage: _____ Cardiac: _____
Diabetes: _____ Infection/UTI: _____
ABO/Rh sensitivity: _____ Uterine
surgery: _____ Anemia: _____
Length of time since last pregnancy:
_____ Type of previous delivery:
_____

Objective

Temperature: _____ Diaphoresis: _____
Skin integrity: _____ Scars: _____
Rashes: _____ Ecchymosis: _____
Vaginal warts/lesions: _____
General strength: _____ Muscle tone:
_____ Gait: _____ ROM: _____
Paresthesia/paralysis: _____
Fetal: Heart rate: _____ Location: _____
Method of auscultation: _____
Fundal height: _____ Estimated
gestation: _____ Movement: _____
Ballottement: _____
Results of fetal testing: _____
AFT: _____
Results of cultures, cervical/rectal:
_____ Immune system testing: _____
Blood type: Maternal: _____
Paternal: _____ Screenings, i.e.,
Serology: _____ Syphilis: _____
Sickle cell: _____ Rubella: _____
Hepatitis: _____ HIV: _____

History of accidental injuries:
  Fractures/dislocations: _____
  Physical abuse: _____ Arthritis/
  unstable joints: _____ Back
  problems: _____
Changes in moles: _____
  Enlarged nodes: _____
Impaired vision: _____ Hearing: _____
Prosthesis: _____ Ambulatory
  devices: _____

SEXUALITY (COMPONENT OF SOCIAL INTERACTIONS)

Subjective

Sexual concerns: _____
  Menarche: _____ Length of cycle:
  _____ Duration: _____ First day of
  last menstrual period: _____
  Amount: _____ Bleeding/cramping
  since LMP: _____ Vaginal
  discharge: _____
Client's belief of when conception
  occurred: _____
Estimated date of delivery: _____
Practices breast self-exam (Y/N): _____
  Last PAP smear: _____
  Pap smear results: _____
Recent contraceptive method:

  _____

Ob history: (GPTPAL) gravida: _____
  Para: _____ Term: _____ Preterm:
  _____ Abortions: _____ Living: _____
  Multiple births: _____
Delivery History:
  Year: _____ Place of delivery:
  _____ Length of
  gestation: _____ Length of labor:
  _____ Type of delivery:
  _____ Born (alive or
  dead): _____ Weight: _____ Apgar
  scores: _____
Complications (maternal/fetal): _____

Objective

Pelvic: Vulva: _____ Perineum: _____
  Vagina: _____ Cervix: _____ Uterus:
  _____ Adnexal: _____ Diagonal
  conjugate: _____ Transverse
  diameter: _____ Outlet (cm): _____
  Shape of sacrum: _____ Arch: _____
  Coccyx: _____ SS Notch: _____
  Ischial spines: _____ Adequacy of
  inlet: _____ Mid: _____ Outlet: _____
Prognosis for delivery: _____
Breast exam: _____ Nipples: _____
Pregnancy test: _____ Serology test
  (date): _____

EXCERPT FROM INTRAPARTAL ASSESSMENT TOOL

PAIN/DISCOMFORT

Subjective

Uterine contractions began: _____
  Became regular: _____

Objective

Facial expression: _____ Narrowed
  focus: _____ Body movement: _____

Location of contractile pain:
front: _____ Sacral area: _____
Degree of discomfort: Mild: _____
Moderate: _____ Severe: _____
How relieved: _____
Breathing/relaxation techniques:
_____ Positioning: _____ Sacral
rubs: _____ Effleurage: _____

Change in BP: _____ Pulse: _____

SAFETY

Subjective

Allergies/Sensitivity: _____
Reaction (specify): _____
History of STD (date/type):

_____

Health status of living children:

_____

Month of first prenatal visit: _____
Previous/current obstetric problems/
treatment: PIH: _____ Kidney: _____
Hemorrhage: _____ Cardiac: _____
Diabetes: _____ Infection/UTI:
_____ ABO/Rh sensitivity: _____
Uterine surgery: _____
Anemia: _____
Length of time since last
pregnancy: _____
Type of previous delivery:

_____

Blood transfusion: _____ When: _____
Reaction (describe): _____
Maternal stature/build: _____
Fractures/dislocations: _____
Pelvis: _____
Arthritis/Unstable joints: _____
Spinal problems/deformity:
Kyphosis: _____
Scoliosis: _____ Trauma: _____
Surgery: _____
Prosthesis/Ambulatory
devices: _____

Objective

Temperature: _____ Skin integrity:
_____ Rashes: _____
Sores: _____ Bruises: _____
Scars: _____
Paresthesia/paralysis: _____
Fetal status: heart rate: _____
Location: _____ Method of
auscultation: _____ Fundal height:
_____ Estimated gestation: _____
Activity/movement: _____ Fetal
assessment testing (Y/N): _____
Date: _____ Test: _____
Results: _____
Labor status: Cervical dilation: _____
Effacement: _____ Fetal descent:
_____ Engagement: _____
Presentation: _____ Lie: _____
Position: _____
Membranes: Intact: _____
Ruptured/time: _____ Nitrazine
test: _____ Amount of drainage:
_____ Character: _____
Blood Type/Rh: Maternal: _____
Paternal: _____
Screens: Sickle cell: _____ Rubella:
_____ Hepatitis: _____ HIV _____
Serology: _____
Syphilis: Pos _____ Neg _____
Cervical/Rectal culture:
Pos _____ Neg _____
Vaginal warts/lesions: _____
Perineal varicosities: _____

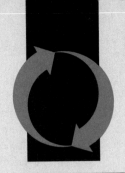

North American Nursing Association (NANDA) Nursing Diagnoses Organized According to Maslow's Hierarchy of Needs and Nursing Framework: A Health Outcome Classification for Nursing Diagnosis

SELF-ACTUALIZATION

Community Coping, enhanced, potential for
Family Coping: potential for growth
Growth and Development, altered
Health-Seeking Behaviors [specify]
Spiritual Distress (distress of the human spirit)
Spiritual Well-Being, enhanced, potential for
Therapeutic Regimen: Individual, effective management

SELF ESTEEM

Adjustment, impaired
Body Image disturbance
Coping, defensive
Coping, Individual, ineffective
Decisional Conflict (specify)
Denial, ineffective

Modified from Jenny, J: Classification of Nursing Diagnoses: NANDA Proceedings from the 8th Conference. JB Lippincott, Philadelphia, 1989; and Jenny, J: Classifying Nursing Diagnoses: A self-care approach. *Nursing and Health Care* 10(2): 1983–1988.

Diversional Activity deficit
Hopelessness
Noncompliance [Compliance, altered] (specify)
Nutrition, altered, more than body requirements
Nutrition, altered, risk for more than body requirements
Personal Identity disturbance
Post-Trauma Response
Powerlessness
Rape-Trauma Syndrome
Self Esteem, chronic low
Self Esteem disturbance
Self Esteem, situational low
Self-Mutilation, risk for
Violence, risk for, directed at self/others

LOVE AND BELONGING

Family Coping, ineffective: compromised
Family Coping, ineffective: disabling
Family Process, altered: alcoholism
Family Processes, altered
Loneliness, risk for
Parent/Infant/Child Attachment, altered, risk for
Parental Role conflict
Parenting, altered
Role Performance, altered
Social Interaction, impaired
Social Isolation

SAFETY AND SECURITY

Anxiety [mild, moderate, severe, panic]
Caregiver Role Strain
Caregiver Role Strain, risk for
Communication, impaired, verbal
Community Coping, ineffective
Confusion, acute
Confusion, chronic
Disuse Syndrome, risk for
Dysreflexia
Environmental Interpretation Syndrome, impaired
Fear
Grieving, anticipatory
Grieving, dysfunctional
Health Maintenance, altered
Home Maintenance Management, impaired
Infant Behavior, organized, enhanced, potential for
Infection, risk for
Injury, risk for
Knowledge deficit [Learning Need] (specify)
Memory, impaired
Perioperative Positioning Injury, risk for
Poisoning, risk for

Protection, altered
Therapeutic Regimen: Community, ineffective management
Therapeutic Regimen: Families, ineffective management
Therapeutic Regimen: Individual, ineffective management
Trauma, risk for
Unilateral Neglect

PHYSIOLOGICAL NEEDS

Activity intolerance [specify level]
Adaptive Capacity: Intracranial, decreased
Airway clearance, ineffective
Aspiration, risk for
Body Temperature, altered, risk for
Bowel Incontinence
Breastfeeding, effective
Breastfeeding, ineffective
Breastfeeding, interrupted
Breathing Pattern, ineffective
Cardiac Output, decreased
Constipation
Constipation, colonic
Constipation, perceived
Diarrhea
Energy Field disturbance
Fatigue
Fluid Volume deficit [active loss]
Fluid Volume deficit, risk for
Fluid Volume, excess
Gas Exchange, impaired
Hyperthermia
Hypothermia
Incontinence, functional
Incontinence, reflex
Incontinence, stress
Incontinence, total
Incontinence, urge
Infant Behavior, disorganized
Infant Behavior, disorganized, risk for
Infant Feeding Pattern, ineffective
Nutrition, altered, less than body requirements
Oral Mucous Membrane, altered
Pain [acute]
Pain, chronic
Physical Mobility, impaired [specify level]
Protection, altered
Self Care deficit (specify): feeding, bathing/hygiene, dressing/grooming, toileting
Sensory-Perceptual alterations (specify): visual, auditory, kinesthetic, gustatory, tactile, olfactory
Sexual dysfunction
Sexuality Patterns, altered

Skin Integrity, impaired
Sleep Pattern disturbance
Spontaneous Ventilation, inability to sustain
Suffocation, risk for
Swallowing, impaired
Thermoregulation, ineffective
Thought Processes, altered
Tissue integrity, impaired
Tissue Perfusion, altered (specify): cerebral, cardiopulmonary, renal, gastroin-
   testinal, peripheral
Urinary Elimination, altered
Urinary Retention [acute/chronic]
Ventilatory Weaning Response, dysfunctional (DVWR)

NURSING FRAMEWORK: A HEALTH OUTCOME CLASSIFICATION FOR NURSING DIAGNOSES

Self care Taxonomy of Nursing Diagnoses

I. PHYSIOLOGICAL HOMEOSTASIS

1.1.0. Alterations in oxygenation
  1.1.1. Impaired gas exchange
  1.1.2. Ineffective airway clearance
    1.1.2.1. Risk for aspiration
    1.1.2.2. Risk for suffocation
  1.1.3. Ineffective breathing pattern
    1.1.3.1. Inability to sustain spontaneous ventilation
    1.1.3.2. Dysfunctional ventilatory weaning response
1.2.0. Alterations in circulation
  1.2.1. Altered tissue perfusion
  1.2.2. Altered fluid volume
    1.2.2.1. Deficit
    1.2.2.2. Excess
  1.2.3. Decreased cardiac output
1.3.0. Alterations in protective mechanisms
  1.3.1. Risk for infection
  1.3.2. [Bleeding tendency]

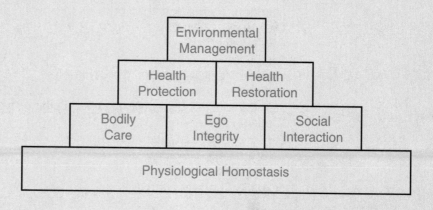

    1.3.3. Risk for peripheral neurovascular dysfunction
    1.3.4. Dysreflexia
1.4.0. Ineffective thermoregulation
    1.4.1. Risk for altered body temperature
       1.4.1.1. Hypothermia
       1.4.1.2. Hyperthermia
1.5.0. Sensory-perceptual alterations
    1.5.1. Specific sensory deficit
       1.5.1.1. Impaired vision
       1.5.1.2. Impaired hearing [auditory]
       1.5.1.3. Impaired touch [tactile]
       1.5.1.4. Impaired taste [gustatory]
       1.5.1.5. Impaired smell [olfactory]
       1.5.1.6. Impaired sense of movement [kinesthetic]
       1.5.1.7. [Altered proprioception]
    1.5.2. [Altered consciousness]
    1.5.3. Discomfort/pain
       1.5.3.1. Chronic pain

II. BODILY COMFORT

2.1.0. Alterations in nutrition
    2.1.1. More than body requirements
    2.1.2. Less than body requirements
    2.1.3. Effective breastfeeding
    2.1.4. Feeding difficulties
       2.1.4.1. Impaired swallowing
       2.1.4.2. Ineffective infant feeding pattern
          2.1.4.2.1. Ineffective breastfeeding
          2.1.4.2.2. Interrupted breastfeeding
    2.1.5. Delayed growth
2.2.0. Alterations in elimination
    2.2.1. Bowel
       2.2.1.1. Constipation
          2.2.1.1.1. Colonic
          2.2.1.1.2. Perceived
       2.2.1.2. Diarrhea
       2.2.1.3. Incontinence
    2.2.2. Bladder
       2.2.2.1. Incontinence
          2.2.2.1.1. Functional
          2.2.2.1.2. Reflex
          2.2.2.1.3. Stress
          2.2.2.1.4. Total
          2.2.2.1.5. Urge
       2.2.2.2. Retention
       2.2.2.3. Altered urination pattern
    2.2.3. [Skin]
    2.2.4. Toileting difficulties
2.3.0. Impaired tissue integrity
    2.3.1. Impaired skin integrity
    2.3.2. Impaired oral mucous membrane

2.4.0. Alterations in activity
  2.4.1. Impaired physical mobility
    2.4.1.1. [Hyperactivity]
    2.4.1.2. Activity intolerance
    2.4.1.3. Risk for disuse syndrome
  2.4.2. Sleep pattern disturbance
  2.4.3. Fatigue
  2.4.4. Diversional activity/recreation deficit
2.5.0. Altered grooming pattern
  2.5.1. Specific grooming difficulties
    2.5.1.1. Bathing/perineal care
    2.5.1.2. [Mouth care]
    2.5.1.3. Dressing
  2.5.2. [Self-neglect]
    2.5.2.1. Neglect, unilateral

III. EGO INTEGRITY

3.1.0. Altered self-concept
  3.1.1. Disturbance in body image
  3.1.2. Disturbance in self-esteem
    3.1.2.1. chronic low
    3.1.2.2. situational low
  3.1.3. disturbance in personal identity
3.2.0. Altered thought processes
  3.2.1. [Impaired information processing]
  3.2.2. [Memory loss]
  3.2.3. [Confusion]
  3.2.4. [Impaired learning]
  3.2.5. [Impaired self orientation]
3.3.0. [Diminished feelings of personal control]
  3.3.1. Anxiety
  3.3.2. Fear
  3.3.3. Grieving
    3.3.3.1. anticipatory
    3.3.3.2. dysfunctional
  3.3.4. Risk for violence
    3.3.4.1. Risk for self-mutilation
  3.3.5. Post-trauma response
    3.3.5.1. Rape-trauma syndrome
      3.3.5.1.1. Compound reaction
      3.3.5.1.2. Silent reaction
  3.3.6. Powerlessness
  3.3.7. Hopelessness
3.4.0. Spiritual distress

IV. SOCIAL INTERACTION

4.1.0. [Alterations in communication]
  4.1.1. Verbal, impaired
  4.1.2. [Nonverbal, impaired]
4.2.0. [Alterations in relationships]
  4.2.1. Social isolation

4.2.2. [Social withdrawal]
4.2.3. Altered sexuality pattern
    4.3.3.1. Sexual dysfunction
4.3.0. Alterations in role
    4.3.1. Impaired parenting
        4.3.1.1. Parental role conflict
    4.3.2. [Impaired work functioning]
    4.3.2.1. Caregiver role strain
4.4.0. Alterations in family process
    4.4.1. Family coping, potential for growth
    4.4.2. Ineffective family coping
        4.4.2.1. Compromised
        4.4.2.2. Disabling
    4.4.3. [Risk for abuse]
4.5.0. Developmental delay

V. HEALTH PROTECTION

5.1.0. Health-seeking behaviors
5.2.0. Altered health maintenance
    5.2.1. [Inadequate self-monitoring]
    5.2.2. [Inadequate self-protection]
    5.2.3. [Reduced use of health services]
5.3.0. [Ineffective stress management]
    5.3.1. Ineffective individual coping
        5.3.1.1. Decisional conflict
        5.3.1.2. Ineffective denial
        5.3.1.3. Coping defensive
5.4.0. Risk for injury
    5.4.1. Risk for trauma
    5.4.2. [Risk for abuse]

VI. HEALTH RESTORATION

6.1.0. Ineffective management of therapeutic regimen
    6.1.1. Noncompliance [specify]
    6.2.2. Impaired adjustment
    6.3.3. [Risk for transmitting infection]

VII. ENVIRONMENTAL MANAGEMENT

7.1.0. Impaired home maintenance management
    7.1.1. [Coping with dysfunctional facilities]
    7.1.2. [Inability to perform household tasks]
7.2.0. [Exposure to hazards]
7.3.0. [Separation from community services/resources]
7.4.0. Relocation stress syndrome

Modified from Jenny, J: Classification of Nursing Diagnoses: NANDA Proceedings from the 8th Conference. JB Lippincott, Philadelphia, 1989; and Jenny, J: Classifying Nursing Diagnoses: A self-care approach. *Nursing and Health Care* 10(2): 1983–1988.

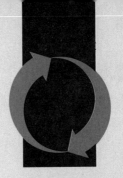

Code for Nurses

1. The nurse provides services with respect for human dignity and the uniqueness of the client, unrestricted by considerations of social or economic status, personal attributes, or the nature of health problems.
2. The nurse safeguards the client's right to privacy by judiciously protecting information of a confidential nature.
3. The nurse acts to safeguard the client and the public when health care and safety are affected by the incompetent, unethical, or illegal practice of any person.
4. The nurse assumes responsibility and accountability for individual nursing judgments and actions.
5. The nurse maintains competence in nursing.
6. The nurse exercises informed judgment and uses individual competence and qualifications as criteria in seeking consultation, accepting responsibilities, and delegating nursing activities to others.
7. The nurse participates in activities that contribute to the ongoing development of the profession's body of knowledge.
8. The nurse participates in the profession's efforts to implement and improve standards of nursing.
9. The nurse participates in the profession's efforts to establish and maintain conditions of employment conducive to high quality nursing care.
10. The nurse participates in the profession's effort to protect the public from misinformation and misrepresentation and to maintain the integrity of nursing.
11. The nurse collaborates with members of the health professions and other citizens in promoting community and national efforts to meet the health needs of the public.

Reprinted with permission from *Code for Nurses With Interpretive Statements*, 1985, American Nurses Association, Washington, DC.

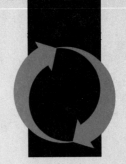

Lunney's Ordinal Scale for Degrees of Accuracy of a Nursing Diagnosis

VALUE	CRITERIA
+5	Diagnosis is consistent with all of the cues, supported by highly relevant cues, and precise.
+4	Diagnosis is consistent with most or all of the cues and supported by relevant cues but fails to reflect one or a few highly relevant cues.
+3	Diagnosis is consistent with many of the cues but fails to reflect the specificity of available cues.
+2	Diagnosis is indicated by some of the cues but there are insufficient cues relevant to the diagnosis and/or the diagnosis is lower priority than other diagnoses.
+1	Diagnosis is only suggested by one or a few cues.
0	Diagnosis is not indicated by any of the cues. No diagnosis is stated when there are sufficient cues to state a diagnosis. The diagnosis can not be rated.
−1	Diagnosis is indicated by more than one cue but should be rejected based on the presence of at least two disconfirming cues.

Reprinted with permission from Lunney, M. (1990). Accuracy of Nursing Diagnosis: Concepts and Developments. *Nursing Diagnosis* 1:12–17.

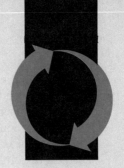

Self-Monitoring of Accuracy Using the Integrated Model: A Guide

1. Pre-encounter data
   a. What data did I collect before seeing the patient? Did I collect enough (or too much) data at this point?
   b. How did I interpret the data before seeing the patient (e.g., relevance of data, priority of data, nursing responsibilities related to data, health status of patient)? What were my biases?
   c. Did I cluster two or more cues, before contact with the patient, as having specific meaning when occurring together?
   d. Was I naming hypotheses before I saw the patient? Should I have connected the data with hypotheses?
2. Entering the data search field and shaping the direction of data gathering
   a. In what ways did seeing the patient affect my initial assessment?
   b. How did I interpret the data that I initially collected in relation to other data, previous expectations, priorities, my responsibilities, or specific hypotheses? How did the patient interpret my behavior?
   c. Did I rearrange any clusters that existed (in my mind) before seeing the patient?
   d. For which hypotheses was I collecting data? Did I consider hypotheses related to the individuality of the patient? Did the patient express diagnostic hypotheses? Were the diagnoses the same as those that were generated by pre-encounter data, or did seeing the patient revise the names that I was considering?

3. Coalescing the cues into clusters or chunks
   a. To what extent did the clustering of cues make me aware of the need for further data collection?
   b. Did I assign validity and reliability estimates to the data while coalescing them into clusters or chunks?
   c. Did the clusters or chunks of data have meanings that can be validated through the literature?
   d. To what extent would other nurses agree with the names that I was considering for the clusters or chunks?

4. Activating possible diagnostic explanations
   a. What data did I collect to support hypotheses? If the answer is none, did I close data collection prematurely? Did limitations in my knowledge prevent me from collecting data for certain diagnoses?
   b. How did I judge the relevance of the data that activated diagnostic hypotheses, for example, were they relevant enough to validate the diagnosis or just predictive? Was my judgment consistent with the judgment of the patient?
   c. Considering the literature on diagnostic concepts, how well did the clusters support the activation of diagnostic hypotheses? Did I consider the unique aspects of this patient when clustering the data for hypotheses?
   d. Did I consider the names of the important hypotheses?

5. Hypothesis- and data-directed searching of the data field
   a. Was my data collection efficient enough to produce high relevant data for high priority diagnoses as well as to rule out competitive diagnoses? Was I able to obtain the greatest amount of relevant data with the least amount of cost to the patient and myself (cost equals time spent, time lost, and effort expended)?
   b. Was I able to interpret the data in relation to many conflicting hypotheses? Was my interpretation specific enough to direct me to precise diagnoses? Was I able to identify the need for further data?
   c. Were previous clusters used, or were they rearranged to produce new clusters?
   d. What diagnostic concepts were considered relevant and valid for testing the goodness of fit after a search of the data field? Were there concepts that I considered briefly during the previous steps but did not pursue?

6. Testing diagnostic hypotheses for goodness of fit
   a. What cues were used to test the goodness of fit?
   b. Were my interpretations of these cues derived from legitimate sources of information: theory, research, norms, and the unique patterns of the patient?
   c. Were the clusters of cues sufficiently well developed for testing the goodness of fit?
   d. Did the diagnostic label fulfill the criteria for goodness of fit?

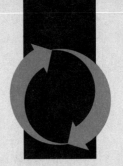

Clinical (Critical) Pathways: A Sample

Clinical pathways may be used as a standardized plan of care or as a guideline for developing an individualized plan for a specific patient. Pathways are best used for acute problems for which there are predictable outcomes that must be achieved within a specific time frame. For example, Donald may be admitted initially to a medical, or step down unit, during the acute phase of alcohol withdrawal. Following is a sample clinical pathway for his 7-day length of stay. After completing this phase, he would transfer to the Behavioral Unit for the rehabilitation program, and a new clinical pathway would be implemented.